SIRTFOOD DIET OVER 50

A 3-Phase Guide for Women
Uncover Your Happy Weight Despite
Menopause and Hormonal Imbalance

KATE HAMILTON

ALSO BY KATE HAMILTON

Sirtfood Diet Meal Plan
A Smart 4-Week Program To Jumpstart Your Weight Loss And Organize Your Meals Including The Foods You Love. Save Time, Feel Satisfied, And Reboot Your Metabolism In One Month.

Sirtfood Diet Cookbook
200 Tasty Ideas For Healthy, Quick, And Easy Meals.
Enjoy The Anti Inflammatory Power Of Sirtuine Foods Combined In Delicious Recipes To Lose Weight And Feel Great In Your Body.

Plant-based Sirtfood Diet Cookbook
Gluten-Free Sirt Foods Recipes for Beginners with No Refined Oil and Sugar

First published in the United States of America in 2021

ISBN 978-1-914370-40-3

SIRTFOOD DIET

OVER 50

CONTENTS

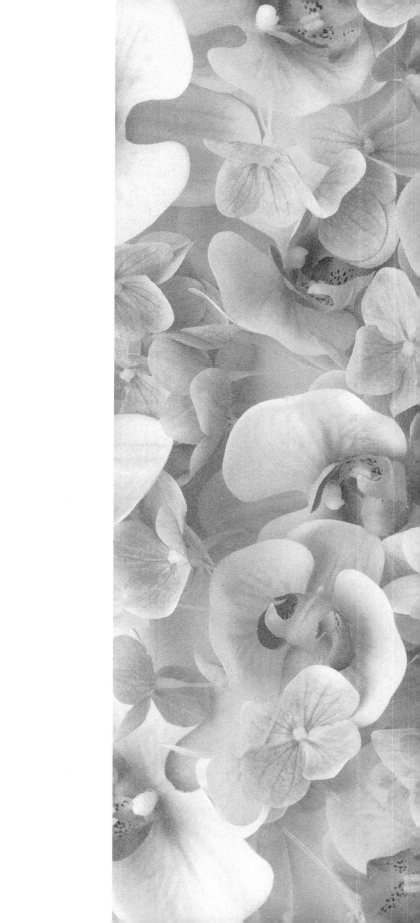

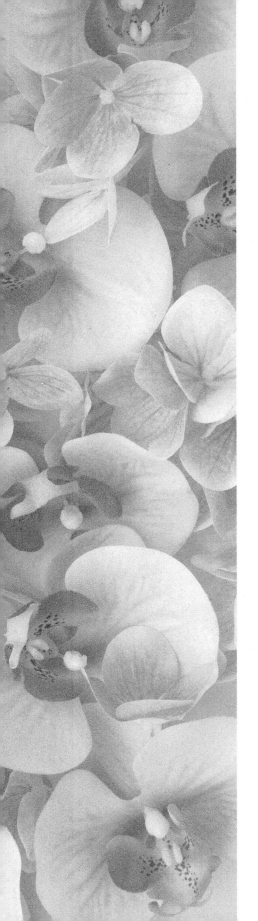

INTRODUCTION

Menopause is an example of how a single word can represent a unique experience for every woman. Still, one thing is sure: each one undergoes a total transformation when it occurs.

For some women, menopause can be light, and they do not feel most of the changes. For others, this particular time can be troublesome.

Menopause involves the end of the menstrual cycle, which results from a long process that begins with the first hormonal changes, typically around the age of 45-50.

Besides that, women can experience hot flushes, exhaustion, hyperactivity, depression, weight gain, and several other issues that may temporarily influence their behavior and feelings.

If you are heading towards the menopausal age, you should take care of your health.

While working out regularly, relaxing, and even meditating help manage the psychological aspects of menopause, ensuring proper nutrition is essential to support the body in this transitional moment.

The Sirtfood Diet includes ingredients specifically chosen for their anti-aging and antioxidant effect. For this reason, it is the perfect solution whether you are approaching this phase, are already in (with all its potential difficulties), or finally reached the stable stage of post-menopause.

The Sirtfood Diet, created by celebrity nutritionists Aidan Goggins and Glen Matten in 2016, is intended to help people rapidly shed excess weight without the consequences commonly seen in other diets.

Some diets require you to starve yourself, causing muscle loss along with fat loss. Others require you to give up foods that you enjoy, making them so restrictive that they are difficult for most people to keep up with.

On the other hand, the Sirtfood Diet encourages you to focus on sirtuin-rich foods combined into delicious and satisfying meals for both mind and body, making it very sustainable and effective.

This Book illustrates a version of the Sirtfood Diet especially studied for women over 50. Unlike the regular version, it excludes famous sirtfoods like coffee, red wine and bird's eye chili, because they are linked to making menopause symptoms worse.

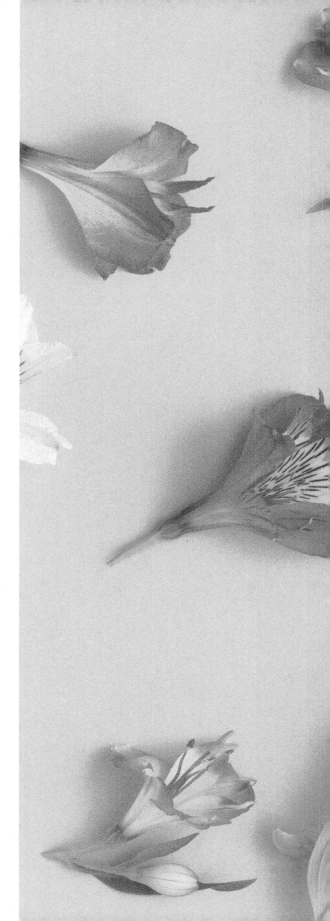

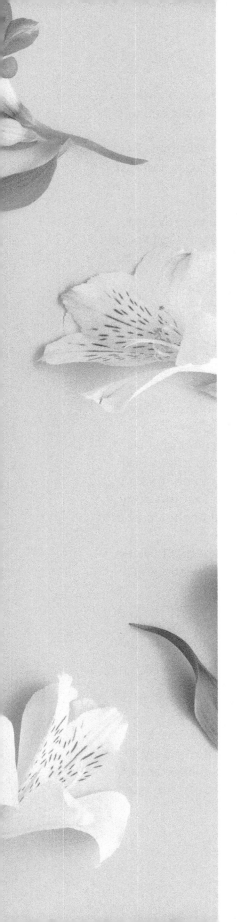

MENOPAUSE: DEFINITION AND SYMPTOMS

Menopause is a natural event that generally occurs between 45 and 55 years of age.

It is defined as 12 consecutive months without a menstrual cycle. It is more likely to occur slightly earlier in women who smoke or have never been pregnant. It is a natural process that occurs because of a decrease in the ovaries' function, which also controls estrogen production.

It is made of three different stages named early menopause, perimenopause, and post-menopause.

The worst is perimenopause, because it is the moment where the decreasing estrogen levels cause the worst symptoms like insomnia, mood swings, and vaginal dryness.

Common Symptoms of Menopause are:

Weight gain
Hot Flashes/Night Sweats
Vaginal Dryness
Hair loss
Mood swings
Depression
Hormonal Changes
Metabolism Slowdown
Decreased Sex Drive

WEIGHT GAIN

Weight gain, specifically a thickening in your middle section, is a common sign of changing hormones. The metabolism is slowing down, and hormone levels cause a weight increase and redistribution of fat.

Preventing weight gain or update the diet to shed excess fat is essential. Fat, especially the one gained during menopause, has been linked to an increased breast cancer risk, heart disease, higher cholesterol levels, high blood pressure, and other health issues.

But controlling weight gain at menopause, while being very important for women, can also be complicated. Crash diets should be avoided, and that's why the Sirtfood Diet, with its mild caloric restriction for a limited period, is the perfect solution to support a gracefully aging body. The Sirtfood Diet is low in fat and high in fiber, primarily from nutritious foods like buckwheat, fruits, and vegetables.

HOT FLASHES AND NIGHT SWEATS

Night sweats and hot flashes are probably the most disruptive of all the menopausal symptoms women have to go through. There are different methods to relieve them, and some of them work better than others.

The area of the brain that controls body heat also triggers the mechanisms to lower it. Blood vessels dilate, heart rate increases, and sweat glands open to release heat and lower temperature. In illness, symptoms often begin with a headache and chills.

Menopause sweats mostly start with a flushing face, prickly skin, and sweat from the underarms. Symptoms of menopause night sweats cause the brain to be 'tricked' into thinking the body is too hot. It feels like a fire radiating heat throughout the body.

This results in a massive rush of heat and sweat that immediately drenches and a racing heart.

Other symptoms include dizziness, nausea, headache, weakness, flushed or blotchy skin, restlessness, and anxiety. The sweats can last anything between a few minutes to half an hour.

Maintaining a healthy lifestyle to restore the body's hormone balance, following a nutritious diet, and managing stress levels are the best solution to keep hot flashes and sweats under control. Substances like sugar, caffeine, alcohol and nicotine are known triggers of night sweats, as well as being overweight.

Sensitivity to certain foods, such as peppers and hot spices, is also a trigger.

This book is specifically studied to adapt the Sirtfood Diet, with its variety of sirtuin-rich ingredients, to respect women's needs during menopause.

This book excludes the sirtfoods less suitable for aging women, like caffeine, bird's eye chili, and red wine, that are part of the Sirtfood Diet originally studied by Dr. Goggins and Matten. Sirtfood Diet After 50 privileges the many choices that provide a powerful anti-aging and antioxidant effect on the body, thus helping reduce the main menopause symptoms like hot flashes and night sweats.

VAGINAL DRYNESS

Vaginal dryness is one of the most common symptoms and also a side effect of menopause. Women may suffer from this in the pre-menopause, perimenopause, and post-menopause stages of their life.

The hormonal imbalance in a menopausal woman causes a lack of estrogen, a vital hormone that maintains the elasticity of the vaginal lining by keeping it moist. A lack of estrogen promotes vaginal dryness or vaginal atrophy.

The problem of vaginal dryness can be very harsh on a relationship with a partner. Initially, it causes some itching or pain during or after sex, but this keeps on increasing even to cause scars and cuts in the vagina, making sex very painful.

Lack of estrogen in the body of menopausal women also causes thinning of the vagina, which makes the walls of the vagina week and prone to yeast and bacterial infections. Women facing vaginal dryness during menopause may also start experiencing pain in the pelvic region as the blood circulation decreases due to lack of estrogen in the body to promote further problems and discomfort.

Because of severe yeast or bacterial infection in the vagina, women may have a white vaginal discharge, which is odorous and painful. Because of growing weakness in the muscles and walls of the vagina because of vaginal dryness, the problem of incontinence may also creep up, and the woman may not control her urine and pass out few drops while laughing, coughing, or sneezing. These problems can make any woman's life difficult, and such issues can be very depressing and debilitating.

The Sirtfood Diet, with its high content in sirtuins, eliminates free radicals, helps to slow down the aging process, and affects tissue regeneration.

Anti-aging is linked to autophagy, an intracellular process that repairs or replaces damaged cell parts. This rejuvenation occurs at an intracellular level. We can't mention autophagy without saying something about AMPK, an enzyme essential for cellular energy homeostasis. AMPK helps boost energy by activating fatty acid, glucose, and oxidation when cellular energy is low. It represents the body's response when facing an elevated energy demand (e.g., an intense physical exercise).

However, a part of this response is lysosomal degradation autophagy. Now you are probably wondering what sirtuins have to do with all of this. Well, SIRT1 can activate AMPK (and the other way around), so it can be considered one of the triggers of autophagy. Autophagy rejuvenates the cell, and this process can happen in all the cells of your body, from the cells of your internal organs to those of your skin.

There are a few ways to induce autophagy, and it has a very positive effect on your health and overall lifespan. Just think of the cell as a car, and autophagy is a skilled mechanic capable of fixing or replacing any broken parts in it. Obviously, the cell will have a longer life, and this extends to your overall life. If your cells are functioning correctly, then you can expect increased longevity.

You can't reverse aging, as there is no such cure for it, and autophagy is not "the fountain of youth." However, this process can significantly slow down aging and its effects. The best part is that it can be activated by sirtuins, especially SIRT1, through the Sirtfood Diet.

HAIR LOSS

Hair loss and menopause are frequently directly related in women. The most common reason why this would happen is that the thyroid gland is not working properly during menopause, causing hair loss.

Unfortunately, as menopause progresses, the level of progesterone will start to decrease. This will increase the production of adrenal cortical steroid (Androstenedione), which contains some properties often found in male hormones.

The result of this is that a woman may start to see her hair falling out or become thinner than it was previously.

One of the typical approaches to contrast hair loss during menopause is increasing progesterone in the body through the right supplements defined by your health practitioner.

The Sirtfood Diet helps to prevent hair loss, whatever the choice to add supplements or avoid them. Hair re-growth though is a slow process, and it may take an extended amount of time to see any change. The Sirtfood Diet supports the body in this transition and sustains hair health.

MOOD SWINGS

The discomfort of mood swings is one of the most surreal emotional states experienced by most menopausal women. While menopause is not a disease, its symptoms often have some women feeling as if they are ill.

The fluctuating hormones - estrogen and progesterone - are responsible for women questioning their sanity and well-being.

Mood swings are roller coaster-like feelings that quickly change from one emotional state to the next with no rational reason. This can occur within minutes to days and can include various combinations of emotions. For example, the menopausal woman might experience a range of sensations that stretch from happy to sad; from moments of complete calmness to heights of anxiety that borders on panicky feelings; from depressive lows to glamorous and flirtatious highs; or from irritability to the most pleasing, agreeable state. While these rapid emotional changes might be related to the low functions of the estrogen and progesterone hormones in the body, women should be encouraged to consult with a medical doctor to confirm any changes, feelings, or conditions with which they are concerned.

Many women have expressed that once a negative thought occurs, all the negatives that had ever been experienced in life begin to surface and flood through the mind at lightning speed.

For example, one woman explained that although these symptoms were not new to her, she would suddenly begin to re-focus on them - such as her hair loss, her weight gain, or her brittle nails. These reminders just irritate her so badly that soon she would begin to feel hot. The excess sweating would then start. The more she focused on these feelings, the more the symptoms became intensified.

While there are various options for the menopausal woman who is experiencing difficulty coping with the emotional symptoms of menopause, first, she might need to check with a medical provider.

Typically, healthy nutrition like the Sirtfood Diet, full of wholesome nutrient-dense food, accompanied by adequate rest and mild exercise, is the most frequent option that may help avoid complementary therapies altogether.

DEPRESSION

The most recent studies on menopause show that 8-15% of menopausal women suffer from depression.

Hormones affect the brain's mood center, and when the level of these hormones drops, estrogen in particular, you experience sadness and a severe mood change, which are symptoms of depression.

Many women that had suffered from it when they were 20; are more at risk than the others because depression is likely to reoccur. Smoking and unnecessary stress are also potential triggers and they have been linked to the possibility of getting depressed during menopause.

A proper diet, like the Sirtfood Diet, is often the first option before evaluating the introduction of anti-depressant medication. Because of its high antioxidant ingredients that positively affect the brain and serotonin levels, the Sirtfood Diet is easily prescribed even during the treatment.

HORMONAL CHANGES

Women who are over 45 years old are the most likely to be diagnosed with imbalanced hormones because the chances are they are approaching menopause.

Hormonal imbalance is the natural consequence a woman experiences after her body has run out of fertile eggs. Consequently, the body stops producing the same levels of hormones, and their lack can cause several issues.

Women with hormonal imbalances may have difficulty regulating their body temperature, retain water, are moody, and often gain weight.

The body will eventually adjust to the new hormonal levels, and it is essential to provide it with all the elements needed to go through this phase.

A woman who is menopausal should privilege vegetables, fish oils, and fruit among the rest. Therefore, once again, the Sirtfood Diet is the perfect choice to support a woman adjusting to new hormonal levels.

METABOLISM SLOWDOWN

Hormonal imbalance causes the body to cling to its fat deposits. You will find it increasingly difficult to lose weight, even if you exercise regularly and cut back on your calories. What you need are some targeted activities to help you lose weight.

Just because menopause is natural, it does not mean that you have to accept its effect on your body. We belong to a generation that fights to get what it wants, and long-lasting youthfulness is not beyond our reach. It is possible to increase one's metabolism at menopause to lose weight and get some relief from its adverse effects.

You can increase your metabolism by getting more activity into your daily routine. Exercise for at least 30 minutes each day without fail since this gets your heart pumping fast, and the effect will last throughout the day. Regular sleep and freedom from stress

are also important, as is drinking lots of water.

A healthy diet like the Sirtfood Diet will also significantly improve your metabolism because sirtuins can trigger the "skinny genes" enabled during fasting, without requiring to fast. Whether you will choose to opt for Phase 1 or 2, explicitly studied for quick weight loss, o opt for healthy everyday nutrition full of sirtfoods, you will contrast metabolism slowdown and finally shed the excess weight in case you have any.

DECREASED LIBIDO

The decline in libido during menopause is a complicated reality to face for many women.

Let's make a distinction between a decrease in libido, which concerns the biological and hormonal aspect of sexual life, and a reduction in desire, which affects the more intimate and psychological side of sex.

During menopause, many hormonal changes lead to a decline in libido because the biological drive to sexuality, conditioned by hormonal factors, is lost. In short, the body no longer finds the "right motivations" to activate the drive to sex, aimed at reproduction, because the woman is no longer fertile. It's not nice to hear, but nature built us that way.

The decline in libido begins before menopause, around the age of 40, and is linked to the progressive decrease in male hormones like testosterone that stimulates sexual behavior and affects dopamine production, one of the most important neurotransmitters for sexual activity.

Another neurotransmitter that also acts on the sexual sphere and decreases during menopause is serotonin, which regulates sleep, hunger, mood and is sensitive to estrogen.

In menopause, the woman's brain responds less readily to biological stimuli, so the time of sexual response is lengthened. The vulva and clitoris' peripheral tissues are less sensitive, and there is a reduced orgasmic response.

Vaginal atrophy is one consequence of hormonal decline, especially estrogen, which occurs with reduced lubrication and little elasticity. These disorders can make sexual intercourse painful, so much so that a sexual approach with the partner is avoided.

Therapies are available and should be discussed with your doctor. Still, it is crucial to keep in mind that no miracle pill solves every disorder, and you cannot delegate everything to drug therapy.

An active and healthy lifestyle helps to better overcome this phase of a woman's life. In menopause, a woman feels less beautiful because her body is changing; she feels less vital, tired, and consequently less desirable. These factors contribute to her being less open and sexually available to her partner. Sexual function is based on our organism's psychophysical efficiency, so an active, efficient body will also be more sexually ready.

Sport oxygenates tissues, increases endorphins and also helps increase testosterone production. It has been shown that those who live longer and well also have more sex.

The Sirtfood Diet supports the body's health and is a good starting point for managing decreased sex drive.

CAUSES OF EARLY MENOPAUSE

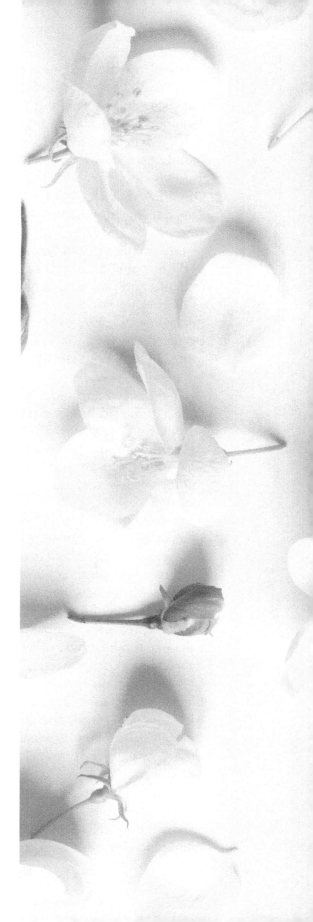

Early menopause, as the name suggests, is the occurrence of menopause before the usual time. Gaining knowledge of the symptoms and causes of early menopause will help you tackle this problem in a better way.

The autoimmune disorder, for example, is a disease where the immune system sends antibodies to destroy the wrongly perceived threats. These antibodies ultimately interfere with your reproductive system and eliminate some of your ovarian functions, causing early menopause.

Chromosomal defects can also contribute to cause early menopause. Some flaws in the X chromosome of women can cause less egg production by the ovaries, causing early menopause.

Women who undergo surgery to get their uterus removed also suffer from early menopause because of the hormonal imbalance created in their bodies.

After removing the uterus and ovaries, the estrogen and progesterone levels decrease to a minimal level, causing menopause. T

Early menopause may also come up as a side effect of cancer treatment. Women who have cancer receive chemotherapy to remove it, damaging the ovaries, causing premature menopause.

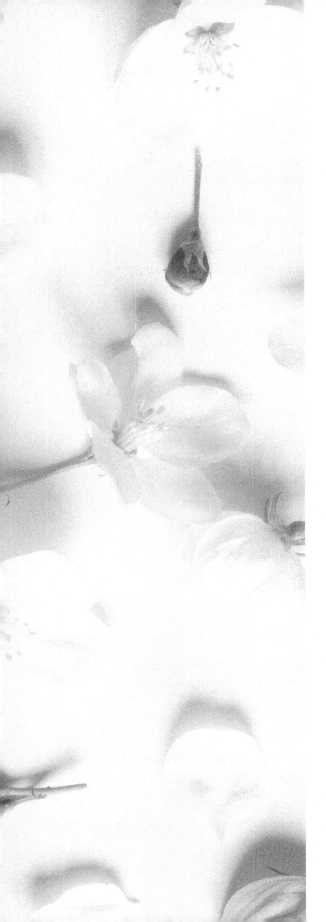

Early menopause can also be a hereditary problem; however, the chances of such a thing are minimal. If your mother suffered viral infections in her uterus during your birth, you might be born with less eggs in your uterus.

Less eggs lead to premature menopause. Certain infections in your uterus may also cause the occurrence of early menopause, and after the disease has been cured, you may not be able to reproduce.

Disorders like Thyroid disorder and Hypothamic disorder, which have symptoms similar to those of menopause, can cause concern for the same. It is always recommended to consult a doctor who will diagnose the right issue and treat you accordingly.

FREE RADICALS

Why do we talk so much about free radicals, healthy aging, antioxidants, and, above all, antioxidants in menopause?

With age and without following a healthy lifestyle and diet, our body becomes a concentrate of free radicals and reactive oxygen species (ROS).

For women after menopause, the issue often becomes even more complicated because they can no longer rely on a team of agents that have protected them for years: estrogen.

Our body defends oxidation through an antioxidant defense system that relies on enzymes and specific substances that act as sweepers of free radicals, always engaged in monitoring and deactivating these highly reactive substances when they circulate freely in our body.

Unfortunately, if we come to produce too many free radicals, our pool of antioxidants is not enough, but there is a solution.

For free radicals and ROS, Nature comes to our aid once again, offering a wide range of foods rich in antioxidant vitamins and minerals, such as Vitamin E and Selenium, and other substances such as sirtuins (flavonoids in particular) found in the plant world.

The human body is continuously exposed to different harmful substances that can form free radicals and reactive oxygen species (ROS).

In particular, these are very aggressive molecules that can occur in abundance in our body because of exposure to smog and pollution, and UV rays, basically different types of physical and environmental stress.

At the same time, we are large producers of such substances that often represent the "waste" of physiological, metabolic processes or accompany the normal anti-inflammatory or immune response.

This happens because we need oxygen and water to live, and these vital substances promote the creation of a pro-oxidant environment in our body.

Under certain stressful conditions, there is a tendency to produce free radicals and ROS. The human body has an innate survival instinct and evolving has naturally sought a solution. We can rely on a pool of protective defense systems with antioxidant action that fights external attacks and our free radicals and ROS's physiological production.

These are enzymes, in particular, Catalase, Peroxide dismutase, and Glutathione peroxidase, and other substances, such as Coenzyme Q10 and alpha-lipoic acid.

To this physiological defense mechanism can be added also the antioxidants that we take with food.

Promoting eating habits oriented to ensure the vitamins, minerals, and other nutrients with protective antioxidant action against oxidative stress, as it happens with the Sirtfood Diet, is the best choice.

The most common nutrients with antioxidant action are Vitamins A, C, E, and B2, minerals such as copper, selenium, and zinc. These nutrients are widely distributed in various types of food, from meat to dairy products, from fruits and vegetables, even dried, to cereals and oilseeds. A varied and balanced diet, therefore, should provide all these nutrients and meet our needs.

As we age, it may be necessary to supplement these nutrients because of potential deficiencies or increased needs. In particular, Vitamin C, soluble in water, and Vitamin E, soluble in lipids work in pairs as "scavengers" in various metabolic reactions of the body and, often, close to the membrane of the cells.

Vitamin B2, copper, selenium, and zinc protect cells from free radicals and ROS, acting mainly as enzymatic cofactors or as mediators in metabolic reactions used to produce energy and oxygen vital to the cell.

Vitamin A is a protective antioxidant specific for skin and eyes. We find it also in nature as beta-carotene, one of the key components of fruits and vegetables, such as carrots, to which it gives the characteristic orange color.

Alongside beta carotene, we also find other carotenoids as pigments present in nature: Lutein, Zeaxanthin, Lycopene.

Lutein and Zeaxanthin, mainly present in green leafy vegetables such as spinach and kale, are widely studied for their protective role in degenerative eye problems, the prevention of some cardiovascular diseases, and the protection of the skin after exposure to UV rays.

Lycopene present in tomatoes, instead, is studied both for the prevention of cardiovascular diseases.

Finally, foods are also rich in flavonoids, molecules with antioxidant action widely distributed in nature. In particular, flavonoids deserve a separate paragraph because they are the main active ingredients of many plants known for their antioxidant activity, including green tea.

One of the Sirtfood Diet's major benefits is fighting free radicals thanks to its high content in antioxidant sirtuins.

FEMALE HORMONES AND MENSTRUAL CYCLE

Progesterone and estrogen form a feedback loop between the ovaries and the brain.

The brain stimulates estrogen secretion through the release of follicle-stimulating hormone (FSH) from the pituitary gland. It enables progesterone release from the ovaries with luteinizing hormone (LH) and the pituitary gland.

These four hormones, originating from the ovaries and the brain via the pituitary gland, form a communication network that regulates the monthly reproductive cycle.

Estrogen released at the beginning of each menstrual cycle, under the guidance of FSH, stimulates the buildup of the lining of the uterus in preparation for implantation of a fertilized egg. In the middle of the menstrual cycle, a surge of luteinizing hormone from the pituitary stimulates an egg's release. LH also stimulates progesterone, which maintains the uterine lining.

Eventually, the ovaries stop responding to the stimulation of the brain. The rhythmic dance between the brain and ovaries then comes to a halt, and the monthly cycle also stops.

This change is gradual rather than abrupt. The ovarian production of estrogen and progesterone declines gradually over the years. During this transition period, the brain does its best to keep estrogen and progesterone levels up by releasing more FSH and LH, respectively.

The combination of lagging estrogen and progesterone and higher than normal FSH and LH is responsible for pre-menopausal and perimenopausal symptoms like hot flashes, night sweats, vaginal dryness, irritability, fatigue, and more.

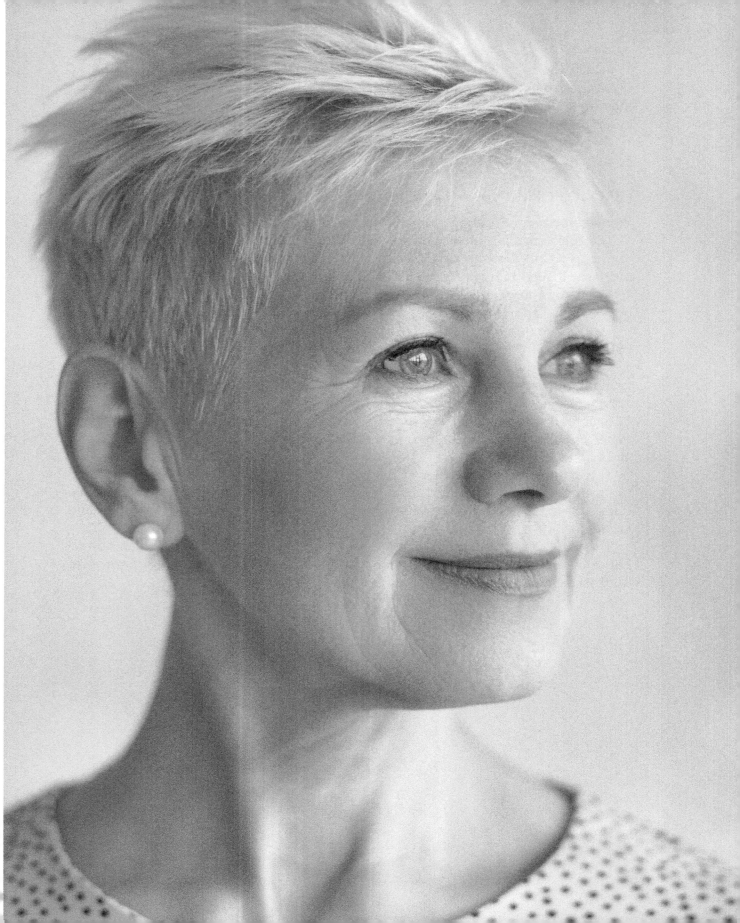

A HOLISTIC APPROACH
TO MENOPAUSE

I believe that the best way to treat menopause is a holistic approach to manage all the points that impact an excellent quality of life after 50.

Of course, medical therapies may be something you want to consider, but they are out of the scope of this book. For sure, either opting to use them or not, the following points are the basis of healthy living at every age. They will help ease disturbing menopause symptoms, like insomnia, anxiety, depression, hot flashes, and mood swings.

Choosing the right diet is very helpful in alleviating menopause symptoms. Eating the right food will help maintain the body's natural balance and being in your best shape.

Increasing the intake of fruits and vegetables and limiting your consumption of red meat and dairy products will create the best conditions to support the body during its transition to post-menopause.

The Sirtfood Diet will be explained in detail in the next chapters.

EASY WEIGHT LOSS

The most obvious of the health benefits is that you will lose weight on the Sirtfood Diet. Whether or not you are exercising, there is no way that you can't lose weight when you follow the diet to a T.

This diet has you restrict your calories enough so that anyone can lose weight. The average person uses around 2,000 calories per day, but during the diet, you will ingest 1,000 or 1,500 calories based on the phase you are in.

A calorie deficit causes weight loss — it is as simple as that. When you restrict your calories, but you keep your metabolism up, you find you will naturally lose weight. This is normal. However, usually, that weight loss is a mix of fat and muscle. As you lose weight and muscle, you would then naturally see your metabolism slow as well.

Of course, this means that over time, your weight loss plan is not nearly as effective as it was supposed to be. As a direct result, you will have to cut calories further to keep that deficit between consumed calories and the calories that your body naturally burns. This means that weight loss eventually slows, or even plateaus if all you do is cut calories. You will lose muscle if you are not careful, which will work against you.

However, thanks to the fact that you do not lose muscle mass during the Sirtfood Diet, you do not have to worry about this problem; you simply continue to lose weight because you can maintain your metabolism at levels favorable to continued weight loss.

Sure enough, one remarkable observation from the Sirtfood Diet trial is that participants lost excessive weight while building muscle, contributing to a more toned body. It is the beauty of Sirtfoods: fat burning is activated, but muscle growth, maintenance, and repair are promoted as well.

Weight gain during menopause can be distressing. Shifting to a low-fat, high-fiber diet and controlling overall dietary intake can help control weight gain. Diets rich in phytoestrogens, or plant estrogens, may offer additional relief. Soy products, such as tofu, soy milk, and soy powders, are rich in phytoestrogens and help lower cholesterol. Linseed products are also an excellent source of phytoestrogens. Regular exercise, for approximately 30 minutes several times a week, can also help control weight gain. Added benefits of regular exercise are a conversion of fat into lean muscle mass, which helps burn off excess calories even while resting. Furthermore, exercise may improve conditions such as low energy levels, mood swings, sleeplessness, high blood pressure, and diabetes.

MAINTAINING MUSCLE MASS

The importance of having and most of alla maintaining a good level of muscle mass is common knowledge, and many don't understand that muscle loss is caused by inadequate exercise habits and age. Between 20 and 90 years of age, we lose, on average, 50% of our muscle mass. Women between 40 and 50 will lose 1% of their muscle mass each year and replace the lost muscle with fat.

The primary function of muscle is to provide metabolically active tissue to our systems. On average, each pound of muscle in our bodies will burn 14 calories in 24 hours. The more we work out and build muscle mass, the more calories our bodies can burn, the more weight we can lose. Conversely, when muscle mass starts to decline, our metabolism declines, and we put on more fat.

In building muscle through exercise, menopausal women can strengthen their bones and help to prevent osteoporosis. Strength training and gravity-based exercises are great for increasing bone mass by stimulating the cells that create bone.

The more muscle a body has, the less fat it can hold or make. This leads to a healthier, more attractive body. Besides looking great, increased muscle mass can prevent some diseases usually associated with age. Muscle leads to an overall healthier body.

Another function of muscle is to serve as an anti-aging tissue. Typically, the more muscle mass you have, the healthier your body composition is. Gaining a lean body can give a younger look. Menopausal women can take 10 to 20 years off their appearance by merely toning up their bodies.

FEMALE HORMONES AND MENSTRUAL CYCLE

Exercise is both refreshing and healthy. Besides, it also serves as a very effective natural menopause treatment. Studies have shown that taking part in an exercise regimen can help ease menopause symptoms in 55% of women. Doing light weight training will help you increase your bone density. Begin with regular exercise that provides at least sixty minutes of movement per day and build intensity slowly.

Exercise helps with body strength and contributes to establishing a hormonal balance, essential to living healthy and happy.

COGNITIVE FUNCTIONS IMPROVEMENT

Sirtuins have been shown to impact neurodegenerative diseases that cause cognitive impairments like Alzheimer's disease. This is because sirtuins help regulate appetite and manage other brain stimuli, enhancing the communication signals in the brain itself, improving cognitive function, and lowering brain inflammation.

Individuals with Alzheimer's have been found to have notably lower levels of sirtuins than healthy peers, although the mechanism of action between sirtuin and the disease is not fully known.

What is known is that the Sirtfood Diet helps prevent buildups of the amyloid-B and tau protein, molecules that are responsible for the plaques in the brains of people with Alzheimer's (and similar diseases that cause cognitive impairment).

SAY GOODBYE TO OSTEOPOROSIS

Osteoporosis is a condition in which the bones become porous and weak. The term osteoporosis means porous bones. This problem is characterized by a loss of bone mass and decreased mineral content of calcium in it.

Under the microscope, healthy bone tissue shows a peculiar honeycomb-like mesh. With osteoporosis, the nests' space is enlarged, making the bone weaker because it is more hollow.

Osteoporosis occurs when normal physiological bone reduction is no longer balanced by sufficient tissue production in question. Bones thus become fragile and more prone to fracture because of the decrease in density and change in their microarchitecture.

The bone tissue, specifically, is composed of a mineral part, mainly calcium, but also phosphorus, magnesium, silicon, and zinc, and a protein matrix, consisting mostly of collagen. In the presence of osteoporosis, both the mineral and protein components are altered.

A slow and silent course characterizes osteoporosis, i.e., it develops "on the sly" and manifests itself with typical symptoms such as pain, susceptibility to fractures, and decreased height when bone density loss has already reached important levels, about 30%.

It has been shown that bone density loss often begins around the age of 30, and the first symptoms occur, however, around the age of 40. A moderate loss of bone density is normal with advancing age and physiological aging, and is not because of osteoporosis.

During menopause, however, for some women, this loss increases substantially, favoring the onset of osteoporosis. Why are we more prone to this pathology during menopause? The strength of our bones is based on the balance of two processes: bone formation and resorption. For both men and women, after the age of 45, this balance is unbalanced in favor of dicrease, so the bones become thinner and more fragile.

In women, with the onset of menopause, this imbalance becomes even more pronounced: in this phase of life, with the decline of estrogen that affects the absorption of calcium, bone density, and soft tissue composition change: the first decreasing significantly, the second increasingly losing its elastic properties.

It's imperative to keep calcium absorption high as we age. The Sirtfood diet includes many calcium-rich ingredients, like kale, spinach, and walnuts, that help contrast osteoporosis daily.

A GLOWING SKIN

Women experiencing menopause are most vulnerable to skin aging problems and are desperate to find the right aging skin treatment. This is because, during menopause, your body is undergoing so many changes. These changes cause your skin to decrease its elasticity and moisture.

During menopause and perimenopause stages, you will have more skin aging problems. This is brought about by the decrease in the level of production of collagen in your skin. Moreover, your glands will produce less oil, making your skin dull.

Another anti-aging skin treatment you might want to consider is progesterone creams. These products are applied topically and have been reported to have excellent results. However, you need to take extra care and investigate its usage for your skin before deciding to use them since progesterone creams are not FDA regulated.

One safe choice is to use a popular counter and prescription treatments like Retin-A. Retinoids such as Retin-A have an established track record of success and help reduce or eliminate the look of wrinkles in your skin.

You might also want to consider anti-aging products that contain lots of antioxidants. They are excellent in making your skin look younger and healthier. If you also want to treat dark spots on your face, try using a lightening agent, one that contains hydroquinone.

Of course, make sure you are using enough sunscreen when you go outside, as nature takes a toll on your skin during menopause. You have to make an extra effort in preventing these skin aging problems from getting worse.

You can only find the right aging skin treatment during menopause when you explore your options. It may take some time, but it is well worth the effort if you want to improve your skin.

IMPROVED SEX DRIVE

Menopause is a new beginning.

First, there is more time: the children are older and unlikely to want to spend the night in your bed if they are still at home with you. Work is no longer a problem, careers have long since taken off, and you can already see the possibility of an imminent (happy) retirement, which on the one hand eases worries and on the other foreshadows a lot of time available to spend among the things you love most, including your family.

There is undoubtedly more freedom: without the risk of an unexpected pregnancy, everything can be much more natural and lived in complete relaxation.

There is more awareness: yourself, your body, your sensations, and your way of having pleasure. There is the maturity to communicate it to the partner - new or established that is - and this makes it even more pleasant moments spent together. Performance anxiety no longer exists, you can feel calm without having to prove anything, and everything becomes an equal exchange where you can travel in harmony and harmony between cuddles and smiles.

This is the coveted wisdom of which we talk so much: continue to do everything but with a positive attitude, a fresh look, accompanied by assertiveness, empathy, listening.

You no longer feel that emotional and sensual drive towards your partner, which can become a problem for the couple. Some women feel they are wrong; others force themselves to intimate relations, even when this is no longer a source of pleasure.

We have seen how the decline in desire has reasons on which you can intervene. Remember that dryness, pain, bleeding, itching, burning, or recurrent infections are not "normal" in menopause and must be treated carefully. Menopause does not mean suffering: many women - for centuries - made a mystery of these disorders, and of everything that concerned their intimate sphere, but today everything has changed.

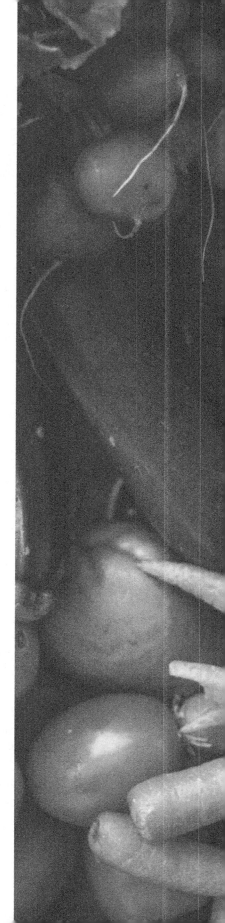

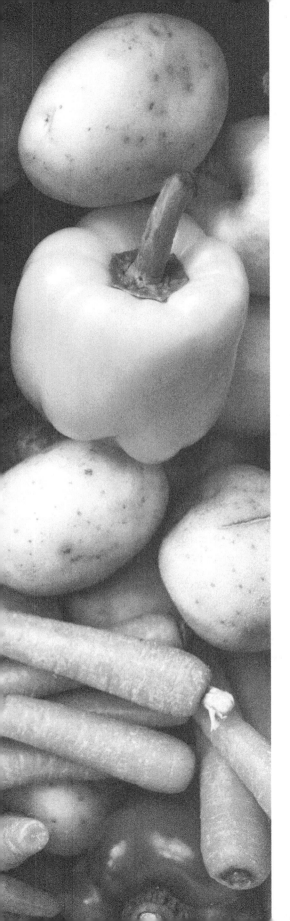

THE SIRTFOOD DIET IN DETAIL

The Sirtfood Diet is very famous due to its scientific benefits and amazing transformations of the body's metabolic capacities. Thousands of people have unlocked incredible and aesthetic physiques by following the Sirtfood Diet.

These results are not coming from myths attached to the basic philosophy of dieting; in fact, the Sirtfood Diet has a robust and growing scientific background. It is essential to understand how and why it works to fully appreciate the value of what you are doing to improve your health and well-being.

THE PROCESS OF FAT BURNING

The most significant benefit of the Sirtfood Diet is its incredible impact on fat loss. Fat is made up of fatty acids that combine to make adipocytes. These adipocytes are clusters of fatty acids, and unlike free fatty acids, adipocytes are not usually present in the blood.

They accumulate under the skin, in muscles, and on different organs. These adipocytes combine to make adipose tissue, full-fledged foam-shaped clusters of visible yellowish or white-colored fat in our body.

Adipose tissue is the healthiest fat to burn, but to do so, it must be broken down into adipocytes first and then into free fatty acids in a process called lipolysis. These steps are not easy as they seem, and burning extra pounds of fats can be a hard nut to crack.

The most challenging step in this cycle is breaking down the adipose tissue into adipocytes. This process is aided by compounds named polyphenols.

POLYPHENOLS ACTION

Polyphenols are well-known chemical compounds that act on an essential lean gene to activate a fat-burning action inside the human body. To be very specific, sirtfoods are foods that contain high levels of polyphenols. These compounds are present naturally in sirtfoods, and, even if they are not equally distributed, all sirtfoods contain specific amounts of different types of polyphenols.

Polyphenols are essential precursors of the fat-burning cycle of the body called lipolysis. During lipolysis, adipose tissue is broken down into free fatty acids transported by our blood and excreted from the body, thanks to the lipase enzyme. Foods rich in polyphenols increase the lipase enzyme, increasing the body's ability to burn fat.

It is fascinating to know that many sirtfoods are widespread, included in both eastern and western diets. We'll discover more about this in the next chapters.

THE ENERGY CYCLE OF THE BODY

The body's primary fuel is glucose, which is the most readily available nutrient for energy. The most significant source of glucose is carbohydrates: carbohydrates are broken down into glucose, which undergoes a series of reactions called glycolysis.

In this cycle, glucose is broken down into energy packets called ATPs produced by the mitochondria, the powerhouse of the cell. These energy packets are used to fuel the body while performing actions. High-intensity work, such as exercise, requires a much more significant amount of energy than typing on a keyboard. The higher the intensity of work, the larger number of ATPs needed.

ATPs are also used in response to stress produced in the body and are crucial for fighting infections. The higher the level of energy in the body, the greater its immune response.

The Sirtfood Diet is rich in low glycemic carbohydrates, essential for fulfilling the body's vital energy and refueling needs.

THE ESSENTIAL ROLE OF MITOCHONDRIA

When a person goes on a diet, this usually means the body will have to manage a calorie deficit. The body takes this scenario as a challenge that requires immediate action from mitochondria - the cells' powerhouses – to produce ATPs, the energy packets to supply the body with instant energy.

Energy can be produced both from glucose and fat, and when the request for energy is very high, glucose is soon depleted, and the body starts using fat as fuel. The Sirtfood Diet, with its short calorie deficit created during the first days, helps to mobilize stored fat and use it for energy, thus causing weight loss.

SIRTUINS AND THEIR ACTIVITY ON GENES

To understand how the Sirtfood Diet works and why these particular foods are necessary, we will look at their role in the human body. As already explained, Sirtfoods got their name from Sirtuins, the compounds they include in different quantities.

The activity of Sirtuins was first researched in yeast, where a mutation caused an extension in the yeast's lifespan. Sirtuins were also shown to slow aging in laboratory mice, fruit flies, and nematodes. As the research on Sirtuins showed effects also on mammals, they were examined for their use in dieting and slowing the aging process. The type of sirtuins in humans are different, but they essentially work in the same ways and for the same reasons.

There are seven "members" that make up the sirtuin family. It is believed that sirtuins play a significant role in regulating certain cell functions, including proliferation (reproduction and cell growth) and apoptosis (cell death). They promote survival and resist stress to increase longevity.

They are also believed to block neurodegeneration by removing toxic proteins and supporting the brain's ability to change and adapt to different conditions (brain plasticity). As part of this, they also help reduce chronic inflammation and reduce something called oxidative stress. Oxidative stress is when there are too many cell-damaging free radicals circulating in the body, and the body cannot catch up by combating them with antioxidants. Free radicals are linked to age-related illnesses and also weight gain.

Sirtuin labels start with "SIR," which represents "Silence Information Regulator" genes. They do precisely that, silence or regulate genes, as part of their functions. Humans work with seven sirtuins: SIRT1, SIRT2, SIRT3, SIRT4, SIRT 5, SIRT6, and SIRT7. Each of these types is responsible for protecting cells in different ways.

They work by either stimulating or turning on certain gene expressions or reducing and turning off other gene expressions. This essentially means that they can influence genes to do more or less of something, most of which they are already programmed to do.

Through enzyme reactions, each of the SIRT types affects different cells responsible for the metabolic processes, organs, and functions that help maintain life.

For example, SIRT6 causes a gene expression that affects skeletal muscle, fat tissue, the brain, and the heart, while SIRT 3 causes a gene expression that affects the kidneys, liver, brain, and heart.

If we tie these concepts together, you can see that the Sirtuin proteins can change gene expression, and the Sirtfood Diet is concerned with how sirtuins can turn off the genes responsible for speeding up aging and weight management.

Another aspect to consider is the function and the power of calorie restriction on the human body. Calorie restriction simply means eating fewer calories. Calorie restriction, coupled with exercise and stress reduction, is usually a combination that supports weight loss. Calorie restriction has also been proven to increase one's lifespan through several studies on both humans and animals.

We can look further at the role of sirtuins combined with calorie restriction by looking at the SIRT3 protein, which has a role in metabolism and aging. Amongst all of the effects of the protein on gene expression (such as preventing cells from dying, reducing tumor growth, etc.), we want to understand the impact of SIRT3 on weight.

As we stated earlier, SIRT3 has high expression in metabolically active tissues, and its ability to express itself increases with caloric restriction and exercise. On the contrary, it will express itself less when following a high fat, high-calorie diet.

The role of sirtuins in regulating telomeres and reducing inflammation is also critical, as it helps fight diseases and aging.

Telomeres are sequences of proteins at the ends of chromosomes. When cells divide, they get shorter. As we age, they get even shorter, and other stressors to the body also contribute to this. Maintaining these telomeres as long as possible is the key to slower aging. Proper diet, along with exercise and other variables, can lengthen telomeres. SIRT6 is one of the sirtuins that, if activated, can help with DNA damage, inflammation, and oxidative stress. SIRT1 also helps with inflammatory response cycles that are related to many age-related diseases.

Calories restriction, as we mentioned earlier, can extend life to some degree.

Calorie restriction, as a stressor, will stimulate the SIRT3 proteins. These will kick in and protect the body from stressors and free radicals, helping the body maintain its telomeres' length. Since this is a stressor, these factors will stimulate the SIRT3 proteins to kick in and protect the body from the stressors and excess free radicals. Again, the telomere length is affected as well.

The research on Sirt proteins shows that, contrary to popular belief that "you can't change your genes" or "my Uncle Joe has this so I will too," simple lifestyle changes can influence our gene expression.

This is quite an empowering thought and yet another reason why you should be excited to have a science-based diet such as the Sirtfood diet, available to you.

PRESERVING MUSCLE MASS

Sirtuins help the body retain muscle mass even when dieting. How does this work? SIRT1 is the protein responsible for causing the body to burn fat rather than muscle for energy, which results in weight loss. Another useful aspect of SIRT1 is its ability to improve skeletal muscle.

Skeletal muscle consists of all the muscles you voluntarily control, such as the ones in your limbs, back, shoulders, and so on. There are two other muscle types: cardiac muscle, what the heart is formed from, and smooth muscles, which are involuntary and include muscles around blood vessels, the face, and various parts of organs and other tissues.

Skeletal muscle is divided into two different groups, named type-1 and type-2. Type 1 muscle is active during continued, sustained activity, whereas type-2 muscle is active during short, intense periods of activity. So, for example, you would predominantly use type-1 muscles for jogging but type-2 muscles for sprinting.

SIRT1 protects the most important type-1 muscles, but not the type-2 muscles, which are still broken down for energy. SIRT1 also influences how the muscles work.

SIRT1 is produced by the muscle cells, but the ability to make SIRT1 decreases as the muscle ages. As a result, muscle is harder to build as you age and doesn't grow as fast in response to exercise. A lack of SIRT1 also causes muscles to fatigue quicker and gradually decline over time.

This is how the Sirtfood Diet helps keep the body supple: providing SIRT1 helps skeletal muscle grow and stay in good shape.

EFFECTS ON FAT TYPE

Not only does the body have more than one type of muscle, as we saw in the previous paragraph, it also has more than one kind of fat too: white adipose tissue and brown adipose tissue.

White adipose tissue, or WAT as it is commonly abbreviated, is the fat made for storage. It's where your extra energy goes, and having more WAT makes it easier to store and gain fat in the future.

Brown adipose tissue, or BAT, is a type of fat tissue typically associated with burning fat. BAT helps keep us warm and contains high mitochondrial levels – the part of the cell responsible for producing energy.

Leaner people have higher levels of brown fat than their overweight peers. BAT is located around the neck and back, while WAT is situated in the areas typically associated with obesity – your gut, buttocks, chest, and hips. By having higher levels of BAT, fitter people have more ability to shake off calories through exercise and thermal release, so although research on BAT is still in its early stages, higher BAT levels and activity is hypothesized as being positive.

Of course, as you might now anticipate, sirtuins also affect our WAT and BAT levels. More precisely, sirtuins help convert your WAT into BAT, changing your body and making it easier to burn calories and lose weight. Over time this will produce substantial differences in your body composition, helping you lose weight and become lean and fit.

IMPROVING THE ENERGY-BOOSTING EFFECT

The amount of energy the body requires depends on an individual's daily activities, psychological factors such as stress, and metabolic rate. Essential body cells and tissues, such as the brain, need a constant energy supply to maintain their functions. The energy-boosting effect can improve the functionality of these vital tissues and cells.

The energy-boosting effect refers to all the activities geared towards ensuring constant energy supply to body organs, tissues, and cells. Following the Sirtfood Diet is undoubtedly one of these, as it guarantees an abundance of fruits and vegetables, plant and animal proteins, whole grains, and healthy fats, which play a significant role in enhancing the energy-boosting effect for a healthy living routine.

Drinking sufficient water improves the energy-boosting effect too. Water is a significant component in every food consumed. Keeping hydrated is essential for body health. Water requirement depends on age, sex, weight, physical activity level, and environmental conditions, such as the weather.

In the Sirtfood Diet, water is a significant compound, for example, in fruits and beverages. Drinks such as unsweetened herbal teas or flavored water are good options for staying hydrated.

Water is crucial in all physiological processes. Thus, frequent consumption of water, and drinks containing water like the ones included in the Sirtfood Diet, reduces fatigue and boosts body energy.

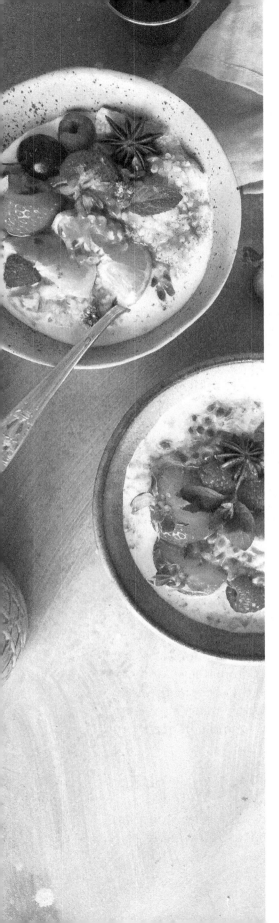

HEALTH BENEFITS OF THE SIRTFOOD DIET OVER 50

There is proof that sirtuin activators provide a wide variety of health benefits like muscle strengthening and appetite suppression. Others are improved memory, better control of blood sugar level, and the clearance of damage caused by free radical molecules that build up in cells and result in cancer and other diseases.

"The positive effects of the intake of food and beverages rich in sirtuin activators in decreasing chronic disease risks are an important observational evidence," said Professor Frank Hu, an authority on diet and epidemiology at Harvard University, in a recent paper in Advanced Nutrition.

Losing weight is simply not enough nowadays, as the diet you follow needs to have plenty of health benefits as well; otherwise, you can't stick to it in the long run. Therefore, you need to see the bigger picture and not focus on losing many pounds in a short amount of time.

Radical diets usually come with side effects, but if you find a meal plan that works for you in terms of weight loss and delivers plenty of health benefits, why not stick to it and make it your default diet?

The less processed food you eat, the more chances you will have to experience your meal plan's health benefits, so you don't have to see a doctor very often.

Let's have a look in detail at the main benefits the Sirtfood Diet will guarantee you for a lifetime.

POSITIVE INFLUENCE ON GENETICS

Is thinness a genetic trait? If so, how can you ever hope to lose weight?

Even if some people are blessed by activated "skinny genes" and can eat whatever they want without worrying about gaining weight, you can activate your skinny genes as well; they are inscribed in our DNA, after all! We just need to remind our cells that it's not science fiction. Our environment and our habits shape our cellular growth and gene replication: this is called epigenetics.

Every one of us has genes able to activate sirtuins or SIRTs. These are metabolic regulators that control our ability to burn fat and regenerate our cells. You can imagine them as sensors that get activated when our energy levels are low. That is the base of most fasting diets. But let's examine the drawbacks of this type of diet.

Many fasting diets have become popular in the past years. The most well-known are the variants of the intermittent fasting structure, such as the five-two diet. In the five-two diet, you fast during the weekend and usually eat during the week's working days. These diets have proven and demonstrated effects on longevity, weight loss, and overall health.

This is because these fasting diets activate the 'skinny gene' in our body. This gene causes the fat-storage processes to shut down and allows the body to enter a state of 'survival' mode, which causes the body to burn fat.

Anytime cells in your body replicate, there is a small chance of your DNA being damaged in the process. However, if your body repairs dying and older cells, there is no risk of DNA damage, which is why fasting is associated with a lower prevalence of degenerative diseases, such as Alzheimer's.

However, as the name implies, the problem with fasting diets is that you have to fast. Fasting feels awful, especially when other people with regular eating habits surround us. It also puts your diet into a social spotlight – explaining to your co-workers or your extended family why you are not eating on certain days is bound to generate doubt and challenges to your diet regime.

Furthermore, even though fasting has numerous associated benefits, there are some downsides too. Fasting is associated with muscle loss, as the body doesn't discriminate between muscle mass and fat tissue when choosing cells to burn for energy.

When fasting, you also risk malnutrition, simply by not eating enough foods to get essential nutrients. This risk can be somewhat alleviated by taking vitamin supplements and eating nutrient-rich foods. Still, fasting can also slow and halt the digestive system altogether – preventing the absorption of supplements. These supplements also need dietary fat to be dissolved, which you might also lack if you were to implement a strict fasting method.

On top of this, fasting isn't appropriate for a vast range of people. You don't want children to fast and potentially inhibit their growth. Likewise, the elderly, the ill, and pregnant women are all just too vulnerable to the risks of fasting.

Additionally, there are several psychological detriments to fasting, despite commonly being associated with spiritual revelations. Fasting makes you irritable and causes you to feel slightly on edge – your body is constantly telling you that you need to forage for food, enacting physical processes that affect your mood and emotions.

Sirtuins were first discovered in 1984 in yeast molecules. Of course, once it became apparent that sirtuin activators affected various factors, such as lifespan and metabolic activity, interest in these proteins blossomed.

Sirtuin activators boost mitochondrial activity, the part of the biological cell responsible for energy production. This, in turn, mirrors the energy-boosting effects, which also occur due to exercise and fasting. The Sirtfood Diet is thought to start a process called adipogenesis, which prevents fat cells from duplicating – which should interest any potential dieter.

The exciting part is that the sirtuin activators actually influence your genetics. The notion of the 'genetic' lottery is embedded in the public consciousness, but genes are even more changeable than you might think. You can't change your eye color or height, but you can activate or deactivate specific genes based on environmental factors. This is called epigenetics, and it is a fascinating field of study.

APPETITE UNDER CONTROL

Though your first few days on Sirtfood Diet, you may find that you are ravenous as your body adjusts to its new normal, but it will quickly adapt to the calorie restriction. You will be okay because the food you will be eating will include nutrient-dense ingredients that will help your body feel satisfied.

We'll explore the complete list of ingredients in the following chapters, but for example, lentils and buckwheat are very dense foods that are featured heavily in this diet. Adding healthy fats, such as olive oil, to your diet will make you feel content, knowing that you have given yourself enough to keep your body going. You will find that you will tolerate the lower amounts of food, which is a huge plus.

PRESERVED MUSCLE AND BONES MASS

Studies have shown that sirtuins can help boost muscle mass, especially in elderly individuals. A study done on aging mice showed that a sirtuin rich diet helped allow for the development and growth of blood vessels and muscle. This would then boost the energy that the elderly mice had by upwards of 80%. That is massive.

If you want to make sure that your metabolism stays regulated, you must ensure that your muscles are there to help you, and if they are not, you can run into all sorts of problems. This means that if you want to find a diet that will help you gain muscle and burn fat, the sirtuin-rich Sirtfood Diet is one of the best for you.

Of course, retaining muscle isn't just better from an overall fitness perspective, but also an aesthetic view.

Another critical reason why retaining muscle mass is important is your resting energy expenditure. Your muscles require energy, even when you are not using them intensely. Due to this, people with high skeletal muscle levels burn more calories than people who don't, even if both are sedentary. Being muscular allows you to eat more calories and get away with it!

Furthermore, sirtuins help improve overall heart health by protecting and strengthening the cardiac muscle (presumably similar to how SIRT1 protects skeletal muscle) and bones. They help retain precious osteoblasts, which are cells in our bones that allow more bone cells to be produced.

BLOOD SUGAR LEVELS UNDER CONTROL

Sirtuin-rich foods are known to inhibit the release of insulin improving blood sugar management. With the use of sirtuins, you can prevent your blood sugar from dropping too low. This is a great point to keep in mind as compelling for completing this diet, especially when you recognize that you ultimately want to maintain stable blood sugar to feel functional when restricting calories. When you limit calorie consumption, you run into other problems, such as not correctly managing your blood sugar. Have you ever skipped a meal or two and felt dizzy or weak? That is the impact of lower blood sugar—but the sirtuins will help you regulate your levels so that you feel strong enough to proceed until you're happy with the result.

BETTER SLEEP

Adequate sleep is essential and reduces the probability of getting certain chronic illnesses. It keeps the brain and digestion system healthy and boosts the immune system.

Sirtuin activators cause the SIR genes to activate, which in turn increases the release of SIRTs. SIRTs, or Silent Information Regulators, also help regulate the circadian rhythm, which is your natural body clock and influence sleep patterns.

Sleep is essential for many vital biological processes, including those that help regulate blood sugar (which is also crucial for losing weight). If you find yourself repeatedly stuck in a state of lag and brain fog, your circadian rhythm may be out of sync. The Sirtfood Diet can help your body regain a healthy circadian rhythm.

The Sirtfood Diet can significantly promote good sleep thanks to the introduction of ingredients like walnuts and chamomile tea, which boost relaxation and the ability to fall asleep easier.

FIGHTS FREE RADICALS

The antioxidants provided by most sirtfoods are great at defending your body from suffering the effects of cancer or other chronic diseases. They are incredibly beneficial for the body — they are designed to protect your body from free radicals that are harmful by-products of breaking down food or being exposed to radiation. Antioxidants work to protect your body against these enemies that will harm you, and because they do that, they can help reduce your risk of heart disease, cancer, and other common diseases that are suffered from today.

Essentially, antioxidants work because they protect the body; many plant-based foods are rich in antioxidants, and they are quite powerful. The body itself cannot properly remove those free radicals that you are exposed to overtime. It is impossible not to be—even the sun will leave you exposed to radiation every time you leave your house. Free radicals and oxidative stress have been linked to Parkinson's disease, arthritis, and strokes. Sirtfoods, with their antioxidant effects, protect you constantly. That's why it's essential to keep their intake up for a lifetime.

FIGHTS CHRONIC DISEASES

Medicine may be progressing, but this doesn't mean that people are getting healthier. It is quite the opposite. Around 70 percent of deaths nowadays are caused by chronic diseases.

This is indeed shocking, but the cause can be traced to the food we eat. The antidote to most of our diseases is healthy food. Processed food causes these issues, but healthy food can make it right.

Modern-day eating habits and lifestyles encourage the accumulation of fats and toxins (fat tissue protects toxins) and increased blood sugar and insulin levels. This is where the trouble starts, from a simple pre-diabetes condition to more severe diseases (eventually, even leading to cancer).

However, the antidote to many of these issues lies hidden within us. As you already know, all bodies possess sirtuin genes, and activating them is crucial to burn fat and build a stronger and leaner body.

As it turns out, the benefits of sirtuins activity extend way beyond the fat-burning process. Whether we like it or not, a lack of sirtuins can be associated with plenty of diseases and medical conditions, while activating sirtuins will have the opposite effect. For example, sirtuins can significantly improve your arteries' function, control cholesterol levels, and prevent atherosclerosis.

DIABETES

If you have diabetes, then you should know that activating sirtuins will make insulin work more effectively. Insulin is the hormone primarily responsible for controlling the levels of sugar in the blood. SIRT1 works perfectly with metformin (one of the most powerful antidiabetic drugs).

As it turns out, pharmaceutical companies are adding sirtuin activators to metformin treatments. These studies were conducted on animals, and the results were simply excellent. It was noticed that an 83 percent reduction of the metformin dose is required to achieve the same effects.

By increasing the amount of insulin that can be released, SIRT1 can help tackle diabetes by causing higher amounts of blood sugar to be converted into fat. So, as the key to diabetes and weight gain is insulin resistance, there is positive news for the waistline.

MAXIMUM FLEXIBILITY

The Sirtfood Diet, unlike fasting, doesn't involve skipping meals to experience the benefits it can offer. Therefore, you are not going through starvation to reach your weight loss and health goals. Nonetheless, the diet involves a brief period of caloric restriction that will require a bit of focus. Then you will increase calories again, going back to having breakfast, lunch, dinner, and snacks.

The Sirtfood Diet has been developed to meet the needs of the vast majority of people who need to lose weight.

Only people with serious illnesses should be careful and skip to the maintenance phase, avoiding caloric restriction altogether. This means that they will still include healthy Sirtfoods (with their weight loss properties) in their everyday meals. While they may not be able to take advantage of the Phase 1 boost, they will still be able to make the best choices for their health and weight loss.

Remember, even if you cannot follow through with the restrictions, there is still a great benefit to be gained from adding the sirtuin-rich foods to your diet. As we will address shortly, many of the foods rich in sirtuins are highly nutritious, and there is no doubt that they are very healthy, and they should be included in your diet whether you want to follow the Sirtfood Diet or not.

Now you are probably wondering, "How am I going to lose pounds by eating three meals a day?"

The secret lies within the meal plan, as it can seriously deliver outstanding results. Depending on the Phase you are in, you can enjoy eating dark chocolate while losing weight!

The average weight loss during the first week is proven to be around seven pounds.

Of course, not all bodies react the same to this diet so that individual weight loss can be more or less, but this diet promises to deliver outstanding results for trying it.

Once you are satisfied with the weight you have reached, you can go into the maintenance phase of this diet and then transition to a regular healthy diet, still full of sirtuin-rich food. Sounds neat, right? This is what's great about this diet — it gives you the possibility to preserve your ideal weight long term, unlike many other radical diets where most people complain that they start to gain weight immediately after quitting.

THE SIRTFOOD DIET PLAN

The Sirtfood Diet combines a short calorie restriction phase with a long-term commitment to nutrient-dense sirtuin-activating foods.

Before explaining how the diet is structured in detail, let's talk about two different and fundamental subjects when trying to achieve long-lasting results.

THE DIFFERENCE BETWEEN DIET AND DIETING

How you eat every day is your "diet," restricting how you eat is "dieting."

Aside from the first week, Phase 1, the Sirtfood Diet is not a traditional diet in the sense that, instead of merely restricting calories, you focus on increasing nutrition and improving the quality of the food you eat.

There are two main phases of the Sirtfood Diet, which are three weeks long. They are designed to set the stage for incorporating sirtfoods into your lifelong diet, eliminating your need to ever resort to dieting again. A third phase is dedicated to transitioning to a regular (not restricted) healthy sirtfood-rich diet.

The average American over-consumes solid fats and sugars, refined grains, sodium, and saturated fat. They also under-consume vegetables, fruits, whole grains, and the nationally recommended intake of dairy and oils.

If this sounds like it matches your current eating patterns, don't be too hard on yourself, you're certainly not alone. You've been practically brainwashed into adopting these poor nutrition habits.

The number of fast-food restaurants continues to grow, as do options for pre-made, packaged foods full of empty calories, and misleading promises.

When you live on a diet of foods lacking nutrition for too long, you find yourself getting sick and overweight.

How many times have you found yourself dieting, starving yourself for weeks to lose 20 pounds? Maybe you've even been successful a time or two and lost weight, but within a few months, all the weight you lost had found its way home again and brought a few extra friends along.

Studies show that when you restrict your calories severely for an extended period, you will gain the weight back as quickly as it came off, and you will do additional damage to your liver, kidneys, and muscle mass as well. Short-term calorie restriction, such as the first phase of the Sirtfood Diet, doesn't have the same effect that depleting your body of nutrition for a more extended period has.

Simply put, dieting does not help you maintain results in the long term.

More to the point, dieting is completely unnecessary. Think about many regions of the world, like Japan or the Mediterranean, where people traditionally don't count calories or diet, and they live to be 100+ with their full physical and mental capacities until one night, they drift off into a peaceful, joyous slumber never to wake up again. That sounds a lot better than spending the last few months, if not years, of your life in a hospital bed, unable to wash or feed yourself, let alone walk around or remember your grandchildren.

You get to choose your future. And it begins with choosing a healthy diet rich in delicious, fortifying, and age-defying sirtfoods.

UNDERSTANDING YOUR HEALTH GOALS

You may have first heard about the Sirtfood Diet because you saw a headline about Adele's miraculous weight loss. Or perhaps you heard that scientists had discovered a "skinny gene," and the secret to accessing it was in this diet.

You want to lose weight, look great, and feel great in your skin.

That is a common and completely understandable desire, but it's not enough to get you the results you're dreaming of, at least, not in the long-term. History has proven to us many times that, even if we succeed in reaching our goal weight, we're either not satisfied, or we are, but we return to our old habits, and the weight comes back.

One of the main reasons losing weight is ineffective is because it has an end or a result that you can achieve that allows you to give up.

If you start looking deeper and making a commitment to your health, you'll find that there is never a moment that you permit yourself to stop. Even if you're relatively healthy today, you maintain a desire to stay healthy tomorrow, and the following year, and 20 years from now.

Health is a never-ending journey, and that is where your real success and results will lie. You won't have a deadline to abide by, and you can't fail, as long as you're taking actions every day that are designed to improve some aspect of your health.

Sometimes you'll see and feel the results right away. The participants in the first Sirtfood Diet trial saw weight loss results within seven days. But other times, the benefits are on a cellular level, and you won't realize they're making such a difference in your life until you're 80 years old and you the only one of your peers that haven't been forced to move into assisted living.

One of the other significant reasons dieting has a less than impressive track record is the type of weight loss that goes along with it.

The diseases associated with obesity aren't caused only by excess weight. When you spend many years eating unhealthy foods, you damage your metabolic system and the hormones that support your metabolism. Issues like insulin and leptin resistance cause you to gain weight and develop even more lethal diseases, like diabetes and heart disease.

The food you eat is the problem, and the weight is simply a by-product of a dysfunctional metabolic system.

If you heal the system by removing the foods that damage your hormones and adding foods that heal and protect your entire body, the weight will come off naturally because you have fixed the damage.

When you try to take the weight off through calorie restriction, excessive exercise, or a combination of the two, you will likely lower the numbers on your scale. There is truth to the philosophy of "calories in, calories out."

However, if you aren't considering the quality of the calories going in, you won't control what comes off. You're just as likely to lose water weight and muscle mass as you are to lose any fat.

If, on the other hand, you commit to providing your body with all the nutrition it needs to rebalance your hormones and protect your health, the weight that you lose is going to be the weight that you don't need. Visceral fat around your vital organs and abdominal fat you've been struggling to get rid of for years will go away, your muscles will be protected, and your body will stay nicely hydrated.

Losing weight due to improved health is sustainable, so you must start to adjust your mindset and your goals if you truly want to be successful.

NOT ONLY WEIGHT LOSS

Your weight is not the only thing you should be focusing on. Your health is the most important aspect of your life because, without it, you will have no joy and, most likely, very little hope of ever being able to maintain your ideal body weight.

If you prioritize health goals, you will have all the motivation you need to stop damaging your body with unhealthy foods with zero nutrition. You will be excited and inspired to try the myriad of fresh new ingredients that will help you feel lighter, younger, stronger, and healthier than you can remember ever feeling.

The Sirtfood Diet is not about taking the easy route or popping a miracle cure pill. It's about finding joy in food and letting that food heal and nourish your body, allowing you to find joy in life once again. There are so many flavors waiting to be discovered; you simply need to commit to making sirtfoods the star players in your diet, with healthy proteins and fats as the phenomenal support team.

You don't have to starve yourself or even deny yourself the foods you love; you simply have to approach food with mindfulness and awareness of its consequences on your body and health.

THE DIET STRUCTURE

Phase 1: 7 Pounds in Seven Days

Phase 1 of the diet is the one that produces the most significant results. Over seven days, you will follow a simple direction to lose around 7 pounds. For the first three days, calorie intake is set to 1,000 kcal.

You will start with a lower number of calories and then gradually increase them. This will jump-start your genes and trigger the sirtuin proteins to do their job on your "skinny genes."

In the next pages, you'll find a step-by-step guide on how to plan your days during Phase 1. This will allow you the freedom to choose from existing recipes in Appendix A or even create your own using your favorite ingredients and the Sirtfoods listed in the next chapter.

Week 1: The first 3 days will include 3 juices per day; the remaining 4 days will consist of 2 juices per day.

Monday
Breakfast: Sirtfood Green juice
Snack: Two squares of dark chocolate
Lunch: Sirtfood Green juice
Snack: Sirtfood Green juice
Dinner: Sirtfood meal

Drink the juices at three different times of the day, as shown: in the morning as soon as you wake up, lunch, and mid-afternoon. For dinner, choose a recipe from Appendix A.

Tuesday
Breakfast: Sirtfood Green juice
Snack: Two squares of dark chocolate
Lunch: Sirtfood Green juice
Snack: Sirtfood Green juice
Dinner: Sirtfood meal

The formula is identical to that of the first day. The only thing that changes is the dinner recipe, as usual, selected from the recipes in Appendix A.

Wednesday
Breakfast: Sirtfood Green juice
Snack: Two squares of dark chocolate
Lunch: Sirtfood Green juice
Snack: Sirtfood Green juice
Dinner: Sirtfood meal

This is the last day you will consume three green juices a day; tomorrow, you will switch to two. Take this opportunity to browse other drinks that you can have during the diet, such as green tea, or herbal tea.

As usual, select your dinner from the recipes in Appendix A.

Thursday
Breakfast: Sirtfood Green juice
Snack: Sirtfood Green juice
Lunch: Sirtfood meal
Snack: Two squares of dark chocolate.
Dinner: Sirtfood meal

The significant change from the previous three days is that you will only drink two juices instead of three and have two meals instead of one.

As usual, select your lunch and dinner from recipes in Appendix A.

Friday
Breakfast: Sirtfood Green juice
Snack: Sirtfood Green juice
Lunch: Sirtfood meal
Snack: Two squares of dark chocolate.
Dinner: Sirtfood meal

On the fifth day, you will ingest 2 green juices and 2 meals.

As usual, select your lunch and dinner from among the recipes in Appendix A.

Saturday
Breakfast: Sirtfood Green juice
Snack: Sirtfood Green juice
Lunch: Sirtfood meal
Snack: Two squares of dark chocolate.
Dinner: Sirtfood meal

On the sixth day, you will assume 2 green juices and 2 meals

As usual, select your lunch and dinner from among the recipes in Appendix A.

Sunday
Breakfast: Sirtfood Green juice
Snack: Sirtfood Green juice
Lunch: Sirtfood meal
Snack: Two squares of dark chocolate.
Dinner: Sirtfood meal

On the seventh day, you will consume 2 green juices and 2 meals.

The seventh day is the last of phase 1 of the diet. Instead of considering it as an end, see it as a beginning because you are about to embark on a new life, in which Sirtfoods will play a central role in your nutrition.

Today's menu is a perfect example of how easy it is to integrate them abundantly into your daily diet.

As usual, select your lunch and dinner from the recipes in Appendix A.

Notes

It is suggested that you should not consume any of your juices, or your main meal, after 7 pm. This is advised due to our natural circadian rhythm or our 'body clock' and how it affects our body. Generally speaking, our body wants to prepare and burn energy in the morning while storing and retaining energy during the evening. Therefore, if you eat later at night, you have a higher chance of energy in your food being stored as fat.

You should also feel free to drink non-calorie fluids. While this technically does include calorie-free fizzy drinks, green tea, and of course, water are better choices. One surprising finding is that small doses of lemon juice can increase sirtuin absorption, so consider adding a dash to your water or green tea.

Phase 2: Maintenance

Congratulations! You have finished the first "hardcore" week. The second phase – maintenance – is more manageable. It will last two weeks, and it will keep including sirtuin-filled food selections in your everyday meals.

The calorie intake for this phase is set to 1500 kcal. This will cause your body to undergo the fat-burning stage, gain muscle, plus boost your immune system and overall health.

For this phase, you can now have 3 balanced Sirtfood-filled meals each day plus 1 green juice a day.

Try choosing healthier alternatives by adding Sirtfood in each meal as much as possible.

You should consume the same beverages you were drinking in phase 1, with a slight change, you are welcome to enjoy the occasional glass of red wine (although, don't drink more than 2 per week).

Monday to Sunday (week 2 and week 3)
Breakfast: Sirtfood meal
Snack: Sirtfood Green juice
Lunch: Sirtfood meal
Snack: Sirtfood snack or two squares of dark chocolate
Dinner: Sirtfood meal

As usual, select your lunch and dinner from the recipes in Appendix A.

As far as drinks, you can have green tea, and other no-calorie beverages daily.

Phase 3: Transition to Normal Healthy Eating

After 2 weeks of mildly restricted calorie intake, you are now ready to move back up to a regular calorie intake to keep your Sirtfood intake high. You should have experienced some degree of weight loss by now, but most of all, you should also feel fitter and re-invigorated.

The suggested meal plan is:

Monday to Sunday
Breakfast: Sirtfood meal
Snack: Sirtfood Green juice or Sirtfood snack (one a day each)
Lunch: Sirtfood meal
Snack: Sirtfood Green juice or Sirtfood snack (one a day each)
Dinner: Sirtfood meal

By eating reasonable portions of balanced meals, you shouldn't feel hungry or be consuming too much. This is the main reason why the Sirtfood Diet is very sustainable. After only 3 weeks, you have changed your eating habits for the better, improving the way you nourish your body. Just keep going, without restricting portions as in the previous weeks and gradually implementing more and more sirtfoods into your lifestyle.

If you continuously try and withhold giving into temptation and always moderate your eating habits, you are bound to crack and fall off the wagon sooner or later. Instead, you should be combining your regular eating habits with the Sirtfood diet principles, slowly aligning your natural eating tendencies and taste with the Sirtfood ideal.

Remember, whenever you need a fat-burning boost, you can re-implement the three-phases of the Sirtfood Diet to speed up your weight loss and cleanse your body.

SIRTFOOD INGREDIENTS

The Sirtfood Diet has some significant advantages over other meal plans or programs designed to help you lose weight and get healthier. The ingredients are very familiar, and you can easily combine them with other healthy foods that are not rich in sirtuins.

Also, this diet is very permissive. You can try plenty of food out there, and you are not limited to just veggies and fruits.

There might be people trying sirtfoods and not losing weight. In this case, their problem lies within the form, variety, and quantity they are eating. It is tough to have a meal consisting only of sirtfoods, so you need to find the right balance between sirtfoods and everyday food.

Having regular meals is very important because if you don't have the meals within a set timeframe, the diet might not work. The general rule about not overeating at dinner or having dinner late in the evening applies.

Over the last few years, there has been an increasing and widespread aversion to grains. However, studies link whole grain consumption with decreased frequency of inflammation, diabetes, heart disease, and cancers.

While the pseudo-grain buckwheat has full Sirtfood qualification, we do see the existence of substantial sirtuin-activating nutrients in other whole grains. However, it goes without saying, the sirtuin-activating nutrient quality of whole grains is decimated when they are converted into refined "clean" forms.

We're not saying you can never eat them, but instead, you're going to be much better off sticking to the whole-grain version whenever possible.

Now, let's try to understand the secret of these sirtfoods. What exactly do they contain that activates sirtuins?

Arugula contains nutrients like kaempferol and quercetin. Buckwheat contains rutting. Capers have the same nutrients as arugula. Celery has luteolin and apigenin. Cocoa contains epicatechin.

Widely used in the Mediterranean diet, extra-virgin olive oil has hydroxytyrosol and oleuropein. Kale contains the same nutrients as arugula and capers. You can find ajoene and myricetin in garlic.

In green tea, you can find EGCG epigallocatechin gallate. Medjool dates contain caffeic acid and gallic acid. Parsley has myricetin and apigenin. In red endives, you can find luteolin. Quercetin can be found in red onions.

Strawberries contain fisetin. Walnuts are a great source of gallic acid. Turmeric has curcumin. Soy contains formononetin and daidzein.

Indeed, all these compounds have the power to trigger sirtuins, but as it turns out, a standard US diet is very poor in these nutrients. A proper Sirtfood Diet should allow you to consume hundreds of milligrams of these essential ingredients per day. If you manage to introduce most of the ingredients and sirtfoods mentioned above into your daily meal plan, you can effectively reap this diet's benefits.

ARE SUPPLEMENTS OK?

The nutrients mentioned above should be consumed in a natural state. This is how this diet works. You may not have the same effects if you take supplements, as the body absorbs and assimilates them much better in their natural form. If you take, for instance, resveratrol, this nutrient is poorly absorbed in a supplement form. However, if you consume it in a natural state, the absorption is six times higher.

Many studies suggest when specific vitamins, minerals, antioxidants, or even polyphenols are isolated and consumed outside of their natural food source, they are not metabolized effectively and, in some cases, can even be detrimental to your health.

It is good to have as many of these sirtfoods as possible to ensure you are getting the necessary intake of sirtuin-activating nutrients. Most of them are very common or familiar. This is the beauty of the Sirtfood Diet: it is not something extraordinary to eat garlic or red onion, strawberries, blueberries, or walnuts. These are everyday ingredients. It is also highly recommended to make sure you include turmeric in your diet, as well.

When it comes to consuming fruits and veggies, most nutritionists agree that it is best to consume them fresh and raw. This is how you will get all the nutrients and vitamins from them.

However, when it comes to leafy greens, another way to reap all their benefits is to juice them. This procedure removes the low-nutrient fiber from them and allows you to have a super-concentrated dose of sirtuin-activating polyphenols.

Since this diet allows you to eat plenty of foods, it rocks when it comes to diversity. This is why you can simply feel free to consume meat, fish, and seafood if you want. As a general rule of thumb, consume less beef and pork and more poultry, fish, and seafood.

The Sirtfood Diet should slowly become your default meal plan. Therefore, you don't have to stick just to the four-week meal plan. Sirtuins need to be in your diet every day of the week, so why stop after finishing the fourth week? If you have a good thing going, you don't need to interrupt it. Plus, the longer you follow this diet, the more health benefits you will experience. This should be the ultimate motivation to make you follow the Sirtfood Diet regularly. You need to check yourself whether you want to prevent or even reverse some of the most common diseases caused by poor diet, slow down your aging process, and lose some weight while doing it.

<u>Note</u>

If your doctor or primary care physician has advised you to take a supplement, follow their advice. There are circumstances when supplementation is critical for your survival. There are many more circumstances when taking supplements is simply advisable.

For example, Vegans are almost always deficient in vitamin B12 and Omega 3 fatty acids because both of those nutrients are most commonly found in fatty, oily fish. If following a plant-based diet is your ethical or moral choice, you may need to supplement for your best health.

MAIN SIRTFOODS TO CONSIDER OVER 50

The following foods contain the highest amounts of sirtuin-activating polyphenols. The polyphenol levels are not uniformly distributed in all these foods, and some contain higher amounts. Moreover, different polyphenols are present in each of them, and they are associated with special effects on the sirtuin gene.

One of the most important aspects of the Sirtfood Diet is to use a variety of foods.

Each of these foods has its impressive health qualities, but nothing compares to when they are combined.

Apart from coffee, bird's eye chilies, and red wine, which trigger some of the most annoying symptoms of menopause, there are plenty of sirtfoods that are perfect for women over 50. These are:

Buckwheat flour helps a lot in losing weight. The overall fat content of buckwheat is very low. In fact, the calorie count is less than that of rice or wheat. As the flour comes with a low amount of saturated fat, it can stop you from binge-eating or eating unnecessarily. Therefore, it can help in facilitating and maintaining quick digestion. The low amount of fat and a high quantity of minerals can facilitate keeping type II diabetes under control.

Arugula is an excellent sirtfood vegetable and is low in calories. It will not only help you to lose weight but also comes with several beneficial properties. Arugula is rich in chlorophyll that can help in preventing DNA and liver damage resulting from aflatoxins. For getting the best from the arugula, it is always recommended to consume this vegetable raw. It is made of 95% water, and thus it can also act as a cooling and hydrating food on summer days. Vitamin K plays an important role in maintaining bone health.

Capers are the unripe flower buds of the plant Capparis spinosa. It is rich in flavonoid compounds that also include quercetin and rutin, great sources of antioxidants. Antioxidants can act to prevent free radicals that can lead to skin diseases and even cancer. Capers can help keep a check on diabetes. It contains several chemicals that can keep blood sugar levels.

Celery is very low in calories, and that is excellent for losing weight. It can also help prevent dehydration as it contains a significant amount of water and electrolytes, which also helps eliminate bloating. It has antiseptic properties and prevents various kidney problems. Consumption of this vegetable can also help in the excretion of toxic elements from the body. Celery comes with generous amounts of vitamin K and vitamin C, along with potassium and folate.

Cocoa, even in its chocolate form, can help in controlling weight. Cocoa comes with fat-burning properties and is the prime reason most trainers suggest mixing cocoa in shakes before exercising. It can help in reducing inflammation and thus can also help in proper digestion. Cocoa is rich in antioxidants like polyphenols.

Garlic is one of those vegetables that can be found in every kitchen. Consumption of raw garlic can help boost energy levels that can aid in losing weight. Garlic is well known for suppressing appetite and can help you feel full longer. Thus, with the consumption of garlic, you will be able to prevent yourself from overeating. Garlic helps in stimulating the process of fat burning and removes harmful toxins from the body.

Green tea is often regarded as the healthiest type of beverage that can be found on this planet. This is mainly because green tea is full of antioxidants, along with several other plant compounds (like theine) that can provide you with several health benefits. Theine has an effect similar to caffeine and acts as a stimulant for burning fat.

Kale is a trendy vegetable that comes with excellent weight loss properties. It is a vegetable rich in antioxidants, like vitamin C, which performs various important functions in the body's cells and improves its bone structure.
It is rich in vitamin K and helps bind calcium. Kale can provide you with 2.4 g of dietary fiber and thus reduce the feeling of hunger. It comes with compounds rich in sulfur and can help in detoxifying the liver.

Dates are rich in dietary fibers and fatty acids that can help you lose extra kilos. However, they should be consumed in moderation as they are very caloric. They allow you to stay healthy and fit, thanks to their protein content. Moderate daily consumption of dates can help boost the functioning of the immune system.

Olive oil has always been famous for cooking food. Extra Virgin olive oil can help you lose weight as it is unrefined and unprocessed. It contains a significant percentage of mono-saturated fatty acids that play an essential role in losing weight. Olive oil is also rich in vitamin E, which is good for hair and skin health. It also has excellent anti-inflammatory properties.

Parsley is a common herb that can be found in every kitchen. The leaves are rich in important compounds such as vitamin A, vitamin B, vitamin C, and vitamin K. Important minerals such as potassium and iron can also be found in parsley. As it acts as a natural form of diuretic, it can help flush out toxins and any excess fluids. Parsley is rich in chlorophyll, and it can effectively aid weight. It also helps in keeping the levels of blood sugar under control.

Endives are low-calorie and rich in fiber that can help slow down digestion and keep the energy level stable, a great combination of elements that can help promote weight loss. Thanks to their water and fiber content, you will be able to consume more volume of food without the risk of consuming extra calories. It is rich in potassium and folate as well, which are essential for proper heart health. Potassium is effective at lowering blood pressure.

Red onion is rich in an antioxidant named quercetin. Red onions can help add extra flavor to your food without piling on extra calories. Quercetin helps promote the burning of extra calories. It can also help in dealing with inflammation. Red onion is rich in fiber and can make you feel full for an extended period without the urge to consume extra calories. It can also help in improving blood sugar levels and in the maintenance of type II diabetes.

Soy can help in reducing your body weight thanks to its essential amino acids. It is rich in fiber that can help you to stay full for a long time. Soy can also help regulate blood sugar levels and appetite control. It can also promote better quality skin, hair, and nails, besides its weight loss benefits.

Strawberries are filled with fiber, vitamins, and polyphenols and have zero cholesterol and zero fat. They are also a great source of magnesium, potassium, and vitamin C. The high fiber content also assists in losing weight. It can help you stay full, which will reduce the chances of overeating or snacking. One hundred grams of strawberries comes with only 33 calories. Strawberries also help improve digestion and can even eliminate toxins from the body.

Turmeric is one of the primary spices in every household. It comes with an essential antioxidant called curcumin. It helps in dealing with obesity, disorders related to the stomach, and other health problems. It can help reduce inflammation linked to obesity. Remember to add some pepper when using turmeric: the absorption of curcumin will be higher.

Walnuts are rich in healthy fats and fiber that can aid in weight loss. They can provide you with a great deal of energy as well. They contain high quantities of PUFAs or polyunsaturated fats that can help keep cholesterol levels under check. At the same time, alpha-linolenic acid helps in burning body fat quickly and promotes proper heart health.

MORE SIRTFOODS FOR YOUR RECIPES

Besides the 20 main foods shown above, you can include many other sirtfoods in your meals. They will help you have a very colorful and varied diet, which will aid fat burning and muscle gain thanks to sirtuin activation.

- Apples
- Artichokes
- Asparagus
- Blackberries
- Blackcurrants
- Blueberries
- Broad beans
- Broccoli
- Chestnuts
- Chia seeds
- Chickpeas
- Chicory
- Chives
- Corn
- Cranberries
- Dill
- Endive lettuce
- Ginger

- Goji berries
- Green beans
- Mint
- Oregano
- Pak choi
- Peanuts
- Pistachios
- Plums
- Quinoa
- Raspberries
- Red Grapes
- Sage
- Shallots
- Spinach
- Sunflower seeds
- Watercress
- White Onions

THE SIRTFOOD DIET AND WORKOUTS

The Sirtfood Diet is intended as a lifestyle; it is certainly not a one-time diet plan. For this reason, it's very important to talk, not only about what you eat but also about exercise. Exercise can act to prevent many kinds of diseases as we age.

So let's answer a common question when it comes to working out, "It possible to combine exercising during the phases of a Sirtfood Diet, or do we need to keep workout routines out of the way?"

The answer is, actually, that it depends.

Especially during Phase 1, when caloric intake is drastically reduced, reducing physical activity seems to be the best option for most people while the body adapts to the changes. It's essential to be kind to yourself and support your body, especially the first three days.

After the first three days, though, if you are already in the habit of exercising moderately, you can start back. It will depend on you and how far you can push yourself. Manage your fitness regime according to your diet regime and to listen to your body. In case you are feeling low-energy or fatigued, stop working out for a few days. Dedicate that time to focusing on the Sirtfood Diet principles for a healthy life.

If you have never exercised before, or you have but never established a routine, it's probably better if you wait until the end of Phase 2 when caloric intake is higher. Then, it will be easier for your body to support proper training.

It is essential to find a healthy and sustainable exercise routine. It should be something that won't keep you from enjoying your life and won't need you to exercise all the time.

IMPORTANCE OF EXERCISING

Proper exercise should involve all parts of the body, allowing your body to burn calories and make your muscles work. You can opt for various physical exercises such as running, walking, jogging, swimming, dancing, etc. As you start increasing your physical activity, you will experience multiple benefits in both your mental and physical. Coupling moderate exercise with a Sirtfood Diet can help you shed extra pounds.

EXERCISE SUPPORTS METABOLISM

The main aim of the Sirtfood Diet is to erase the extra pounds from your body. Staying inactive can result in obesity and weight gain. To understand the overall effect exercise has on weight reduction, you need a clear understanding of the relationship between energy expenditure and exercise.

The human body expends energy in three ways: exercise, digestion, and the maintenance of body functions, such as breathing and heart rate. The diet begins with calorie reduction, and which can lower the metabolism. This might result in slowed weight loss. On the other hand, exercising along with your diet plan can improve the metabolic rate, helping you burn more calories. Thus, you will be able to lose more weight without affecting your muscle mass.

It has been found that the combination of aerobic exercise and resistance training can improve fat loss and can also help in the maintenance of muscle mass. So, make sure that you opt for moderate exercise as soon as you can, preferably before the end of Phase 2.

EXERCISE CAN SUPPORT YOUR MOOD

Exercise can help uplift your mood. It can also help you deal with depression, stress, and anxiety. As you begin the Sirtfood Diet, your body will enter a state of shock during the first few days due to the sudden calorie restriction. Moderate exercise can help you deal with this kind of stress. Exercising causes specific changes in the brain that can regulate anxiety and stress. It can also improve the brain's sensitivity to hormones such as norepinephrine and serotonin, which help relieve depression.

Also, exercising can improve endorphins production, which promotes positive feelings, helping people who suffer from anxiety. With moderate exercise, you will become more aware of your mental state. It does not matter how intensively you exercise; you will benefit even from moderate exercise. As you cut down calories during the first phase of the diet, you will most likely experience mood swings. If you feel strong enough, exercise can play a profound role in regulating your mood, especially during this phase.

EXERCISE IMPROVES ENERGY LEVELS

Exercise has the incredible power of boosting your energy levels. If you suffer from a medical condition, it can help improve your energy as well. While on the Sirtfood Diet, energy is provided by the body by burning body fat. When you couple it with proper exercise, you can improve the benefits. Exercise can boost the energy levels also of CFS, or chronic fatigue syndrome, sufferers.

EXERCISE CAN REDUCE CHRONIC DISEASES

A chronic lack of physical activity can lead to chronic diseases. Regular exercise can improve sensitivity to insulin, body composition, and also cardiovascular fitness. It can also help maintain blood pressure and body fat levels.

Lack of physical exercise, even for a short period, can result in the development of body fat and can also increase the overall risk of developing type II diabetes. Physical exercise must be combined with a proper diet to reduce belly fat.

EXERCISING IS BENEFICIAL FOR BONES AND MUSCLES

Exercise can play a beneficial role in maintaining and building strong bones and muscles. Different types of physical activity, such as weight lifting, can help build muscles when coupled with proper protein intake. This is mainly because exercise helps release certain hormones that can promote the muscles' capability to absorb amino acids. This ultimately helps grow muscles and reduce their breakdown. As our bodies age, we tend to lose muscle mass along with muscle function. This can result in disabilities and injuries. It is essential to opt for daily physical activity to retain muscle mass while following a diet. It can help maintain your strength with age.

Exercising can improve bone density and help prevent osteoporosis later in life. Studies show that high impact exercise, such as running and gymnastics, or sports such as basketball and soccer, improve bone density at higher rates than non-impact activities, such as cycling and swimming.

IMPROVES SKIN HEALTH

Skin quality is affected by high amounts of oxidative stress on the body. Oxidative stress occurs when the body's antioxidant defenses cannot mend the damage caused to cells. Exhausting and intense physical activity can also result in oxidative damage; moderate daily exercise, on the other hand, can improve the production of antioxidants naturally. This can help protect skin cells. Similarly, exercise can help stimulate blood flow and induce adaptations of the skin cells that delay skin aging.

IMPROVES MEMORY AND HEALTH

It has been found that brain function can be improved with the help of regular exercise. Exercise can also help protect your memory and cognition since it improves blood circulation to the brain. Regular exercise with a proper diet is even more critical for older adults as increased rates of inflammation and oxidative stress linked to aging can also lead to changes in brain structure and function. **Exercise Can Improve Sleep Quality** Regular exercise with a balanced diet can help you relax and sleep well because they help release stress and increase body temperature directly related to sleep quality. Exercising can help with sleep disorders, as well. You can be completely flexible regarding the type of exercise that you want to choose. The best results have been shown with aerobic exercise, coupled with resistance training.

EXERCISE CAN HELP REDUCE PAIN

Chronic pain can be debilitating. But, with the help of exercise, you can deal with it very easily. Exercise helps tone the muscles that remain inactive, which, in turn, results in the reduction of pain. You will be able to improve your level of pain tolerance and decrease pain perception with daily exercise.

FITNESS OVER 50

Many people think that getting older means they have fewer worries and can relax. After all, children have grown up, and responsibilities have decreased. If you also think so, you should know that the absence of exercise has serious consequences: reduction in cognitive abilities, loss of muscle mass, tone, and flexibility, loss of movement capacity. reduction in agility, in moving from one point to another.
If you are one of those people who take care of themselves, the effects just mentioned will not please you one bit.
Here, a few reccomendations when exercising after 50.

Do not neglect physical pain
You will have heard for sure that "if it hurts, it means it works." Many people believe that exercise must cause some type of pain to show its effects.
In reality, this is not the case. If you notice pain, you need to see if it is constant or if it occurs when you are doing certain activities.
Exercising after the age of 50 implies taking specific precautionary measures; one of them is changing sports.
If, for example, you suffer from the onset of osteoporosis; you need to change the exercises you do, switching to less intense training. Instead of going out for a run, walk, or do yoga.
In case your lifestyle has always been healthy and full of exercise, just pay attention to the changes you might have to implement; one of them could reduce your speed.
You don't have to worry: it's just your body changing.

Don't neglect your back health

Have you always been a fan of rock climbing or other extreme sports? If so, know that practicing these sports after 50 can mean back pain if you don't change your sport.

Unfortunately, your body is changing, so it is highly recommended that you leave certain sports aside.

This is not always the case, but your spine may send you signals.

You don't need to implement these changes in most cases, but if you neglected stretching or warming up in your youth, you will now notice the consequences of this carelessness.

Pamper yourself!

After a good workout session, take a deep breath and pamper your body. You have several options to choose from:

Take a shower with warm water to relax. It is perfect to avoid pain and discomfort the next day. If you started exercising after the age of 50, after years of inactivity, this trick is especially recommended.

Few things are as pleasant as taking a bath surrounded by a pleasant scent. Take some time to enjoy this moment and get in touch with your body. You might take the opportunity to get a massage if you're feeling tense.

Avoid a sedentary life

Whatever sport you choose, the important thing is that you do physical activity.

Don't let yourself go! Exercising after 50, when you once had a routine full of work and family commitments, may make you feel sluggish.

Yet, sitting in a chair will make you feel unproductive and even depressed. For this reason, we recommend that you:

Walk.

Visit family or friends.

Visit and explore unknown places.

Do not hesitate

Just because you want to exercise after age 50 and have more free time than before doesn't mean you have to overdo it. Try to incorporate fun activities into your daily routine instead of planning a 3-hour workout. Don't tell yourself that exercising after 50 is useless. If you've spent your life avoiding physical activity, chances are you think you don't need it. Abandon this thought altogether and find the drive to lead a healthier life. There are many good reasons to do so, but the important thing is to be healthy and independent.

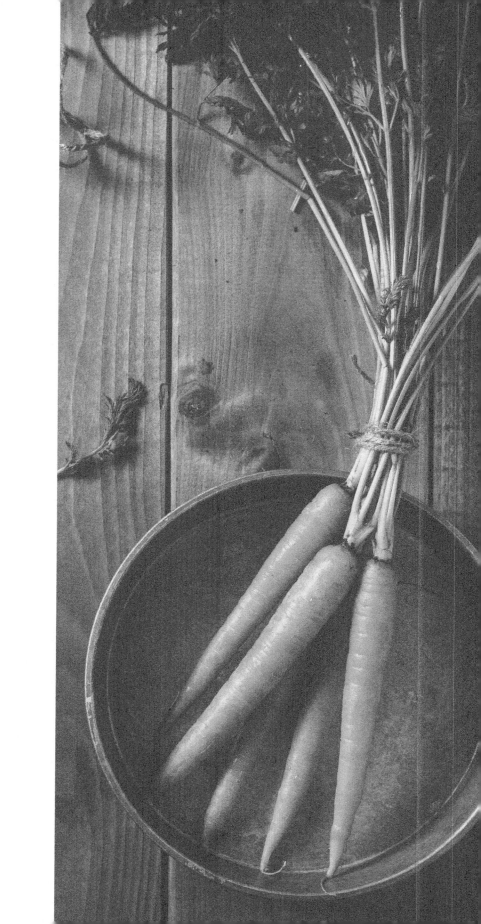

CONCLUSION

The fertile season of a woman's life ends when she enters menopause.

This is a physiological condition - therefore absolutely normal - and that does not occur suddenly but gradually, in an interval that varies from a few months to a few years. The progressive decline of ovarian function accompanies that. This period is called perimenopause and can bring a series of discomfort and disorders, such as hot flashes, sweating, and irritability.

These manifestations are the consequence of the dancing hormones: estrogen and progesterone levels fall until they disappear, putting out of order the brain's central unit (hypothalamus) that regulates all our biorhythms. In fact, in this first period, all symptoms are felt with greater intensity.

The actual menopause arrives when more than a year has passed since the last menstruation, on average between 46 and 55 years. The good news is that in this phase, after reaching the peak, usually your ailments slowly decrease in intensity and subside their incidence in daily life.

The Sirtfood Diet is an effective nutrition plan that can help a woman during her transition to post-menopause. It is a lifestyle change that can be done without effort and allows you to enjoy the anti-aging benefits of sirtuins for a lifetime.

Eat better to live better, with the Sirtfood Diet After 50.

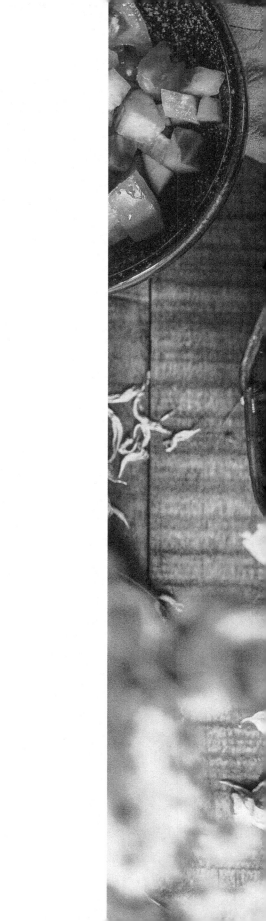

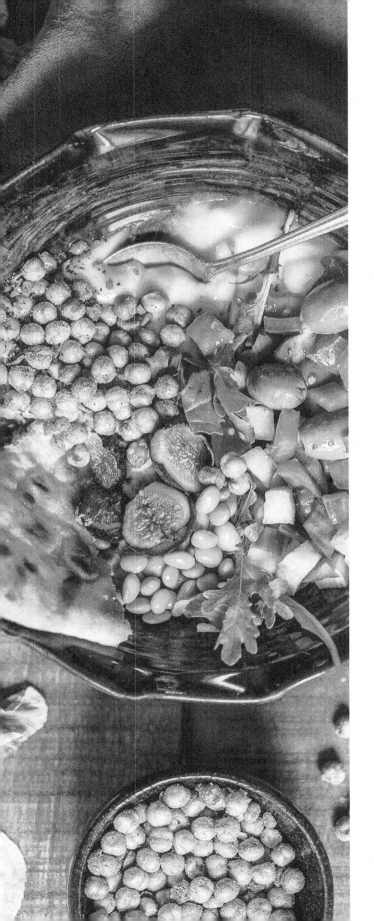

APPENDICES

APPENDIX A

SIRTFOOD RECIPES

BREAKFAST

SIRTFOOD GREEN JUICE

 1   5 mins

Ingredients:
  Recipe 1:
    1 tbsp. parsley
    1 stalk celery
    1 apple
    ½ lemon
  Recipe 2:
    1 cucumber
    1 stalk celery
    1 apple
    3 mint leaves

Directions:
Choose one of the recipes.

Add all ingredients into a juicer and extract the juice according to the manufacturer's method.

In case you don't have one, add all the ingredients in a blender and pulse until well combined.

Filter the juice through a fine-mesh strainer and transfer it into a glass. Top with water if needed. Serve immediately.

NUTRITION FACTS: CALORIES 30KCAL FAT 0.4 G CARBOHYDRATE 4.5 G PROTEIN 1 G

CHOCOLATE DESSERT WITH DATES AND WALNUTS

 2   🕐 25 mins

Ingredients:
4 Medjool dates, pitted
2 tbsp. cocoa powder
1 cup milk, skimmed
1 tsp. agar powder
1 tbsp. peanut butter
1 pinch of salt
½ tsp. cinnamon
2 walnuts
1 tsp whole wheat flour

Directions:
Blitz dates, peanut butter, and 1 tbsp. milk in a food processor.

Put the mix in a pan; add cocoa, cinnamon, salt, flour, agar powder. Add the remaining hot milk bit by bit and mix well to obtain a smooth mixture.

Turn the heat on, bring to a boil and cook around 6-8 minutes until dense. Divide into 2 cups, let cool, and put in the fridge. Add chopped walnuts before serving.

NUTRITION FACTS: CALORIES 326KCAL FAT 3 G CARBOHYDRATE 7 G PROTEIN 25 G

PANCAKES WITH CARAMELIZED STRAWBERRIES

🥘 2   🕐 20 mins

Ingredients:
1 egg
1 ½ oz. self-raising flour
1 ½ oz. buckwheat flour
1/3 cup skimmed milk
1 cup strawberries
2 tsp honey

Directions:
Mix the flours in a bowl; add the yolk and form a very thick batter. Keep adding the milk bit by bit to avoid lumps.

In another bowl, beat the egg white until stiff and then mix it carefully into the batter.

Pour enough batter to make a 5-inch round pancake and cook 2 minutes per side until done. Repeat until all the pancakes are ready.

Put strawberries and honey in a hot pan until caramelized, then put half of the strawberry and honey mixture on top of each pancake serving.

NUTRITION FACTS: CALORIES 272KCAL FAT 4.3 G CARBOHYDRATE 26.8 G PROTEIN 23.6 G

MATCHA OVERNIGHT OATS

 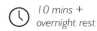 2   10 mins + overnight rest

Ingredients:
2 tsp. chia seeds
3 oz. rolled oats
1 tsp. matcha powder
1 tsp honey
1 ½ cups almond milk
2 pinches ground cinnamon
1 apple, peeled, cored, and chopped
4 walnuts

NUTRITION FACTS: CALORIES 324KCAL FAT 4 G CARBOHYDRATE 37 G PROTEIN 22 G

Directions:
Place the chia seeds and the oats in a container or bowl.

In a different jug or bowl, add the matcha powder and one tablespoon of almond milk and whisk with a hand-held mixer until you get a smooth paste, then add the rest of the milk and mix thoroughly.

Pour the milk mixture over the oats, add the honey and cinnamon, and then stir well. Cover the bowl with a lid and place in the fridge overnight.

When you want to eat, transfer the oats to two serving bowls, top with the walnuts and chopped apple.

SCRAMBLED EGGS AND RED ONION

  1   4 mins

Ingredients:
2 eggs
1 tbsp. parmesan
Salt and pepper
½ cup red onion
1 tbsp. parsley, finely chopped

Directions:
Put eggs and cheese with a pinch of salt and pepper and finely chopped onion in a bowl. Whisk quickly.

Cook the scrambled eggs in a skillet for 2 minutes, stirring continuously until done.

NUTRITION FACTS: CALORIES 278KCAL FAT 5.4 G CARBOHYDRATE 12.8 G PROTEIN 18.9 G

WALNUT DATE BANANA BREAD

 8   *30 mins*

Ingredients:
¾ cup whole-wheat flour
¼ cup buckwheat flour
1 tbsp. cinnamon
½ tbsp. salt
¼ tbsp. baking soda
2 medium, ripe bananas, mashed
2 eggs, gently beaten
½ cup granulated sugar
⅓ cup plain nonfat yogurt
2 tbsp. vegetable oil
1 tbsp. vanilla concentrate
2 tbsp. toasted pecans, chopped
½ cups walnuts, chopped
4 dates, chopped

Directions:
Mix flour with cinnamon, baking soda, and salt in a bowl. In another bowl, whisk together bananas, eggs, sugar, yogurt, oil, and vanilla. Add flour to a greased loaf baking pan and sprinkle walnuts and dates on top.

Heat the oven to 310°F, and cook 30 to 35 minutes. Always check with a stick if the bread is well cooked through (prick the bread with the stick, that has to stay dry).

Move bread to a wire rack to cool before cutting it.

NUTRITION FACTS: CALORIES 180KCAL FAT 6 G CARBOHYDRATE 29 G PROTEIN 4 G

AIR FRIED CHICKEN WITH SALAD SPROUTS

 1   🕐 30 mins

Ingredients:
8 oz. chicken breasts
⅛ tbsp. salt
½ tbsp. pepper,
1 tbsp. extra-virgin olive oil
1 tbsp. maple syrup
1 tbsp. Dijon mustard
6 oz. Brussels sprouts
1 garlic clove, crushed
1 handful parsley, chopped

Directions:
Spray the chicken breast with cooking spray; sprinkle with salt and 1/4 tbsp. of the pepper.

Whisk together oil, maple syrup, mustard, and 1/4 tbsp. pepper in a bowl. Add Brussels sprouts; toss to cover.

Put the chicken breast on one side of a pan, and add Brussels sprouts on the other.

Heat the oven (or air fryer) to 400°F and cook until the chicken is well colored and cooked through (15 to 18 minutes).

NUTRITION FACTS: CALORIES 337KCAL FAT 7 G CARBOHYDRATE 21 G PROTEIN 25 G

AROMATIC CURRY

 4   🕐 40 mins

Ingredients:

19 oz. garbanzo beans
2 cup vegetable broth
10 oz. spinach
7 garlic cloves, diced
3 red onions, diced
2 carrots, chopped
2 tsp. ground cumin
1 handful parsley, chopped
1 tsp. turmeric
1 tbsp. paprika
2 tsp. salt
1 tsp. ground black pepper
1/4 tsp. ginger, grated
1 yellow bell pepper, chopped
3 tbsp. extra-virgin olive oil
⅔ cup coconut milk
½ cup slivered almonds
½ cup golden raisins
2 cups cooked rice

Directions:

In a saucepan, add the spinach and cook on low heat, allowing it to thaw. Sautè garlic, onions in another pan with oil on medium.

Add the carrots and cook for 4 to 6 minutes, until the onions are golden brown.

Add the raisins, garbanzo beans, cumin, turmeric, ginger, paprika, and parsley and cook for 2 minutes.

Add the spinach, bell pepper, broth, and coconut milk, reduce heat to low, and simmer, covered, for 30 minutes.

Serve hot with rice.

NUTRITION FACTS: CALORIES 316KCAL FAT 5.2 G CARBOHYDRATE 13.1 G PROTEIN 6.9 G

ASIAN CHICKEN DRUMSTICKS

 2   🕐 36 mins

Ingredients:

6 chicken drumsticks
¼ cup rice vinegar
3 tbsp. agave syrup
2 tbsp. chicken stock
1 tbsp. lower-sodium soy sauce
1 tbsp. sesame oil
1 tbsp. tomato paste
1 garlic clove, crushed
2 tbsp. walnuts, chopped
½ tsp. turmeric

Directions:

Put the chicken in a single layer in the oven and cook at 400°F until the skin is crispy (around 25 to 28 minutes), turning drumsticks over partway through cooking.

In the meantime, mix vinegar, stock, agave, soy sauce, oil, tomato paste, and garlic in a skillet.

Bring to a boil over medium-high. Cook for about 6 minutes until thickened.

Put the drumsticks and sauce in a bowl and toss to cover. Sprinkle with walnuts.

NUTRITION FACTS: CALORIES 388KCAL FAT 10 G CARBOHYDRATES 20 G PROTEIN 25 G

CHICKEN KOFTE WITH ZUCCHINI

🍲 4   🕐 52 mins

Ingredients:

½ cup low-fat Greek yogurt
2 tbsp. black olives, pitted and chopped
1 handful parsley, chopped
¼ cup breadcrumbs
½ red onion, cubed
1 tbsp. ground cumin
1-pound ground chicken
4 tbsp. olive oil
4 zucchini, sliced

Directions:

Mix yogurt, black olives, parsley, breadcrumbs, onion, 1/2 tbsp. salt, and 1/4 tbsp. pepper in a bowl, mixing with a whisk.

Add chicken; blend in with hands. Shape chicken mixture into 8 patties. Heat 2 tbsp. olive oil in a skillet over medium heat. Add patties; cook 4 minutes on each side or until done.

While kofte cooks, cook zucchini on a skillet. Brush them with 2 tbsp oil and season with the remaining pepper.

Cook on high heat for 5 minutes, then season with salt. Serve 2 kofte per person with zucchini on the side.

NUTRITION FACTS: CALORIES 301KCAL FAT 6.9 G CARBOHYDRATE 15 G PROTEIN 24 G

SIRT CHICKEN SOUVLAKI

 4   🕐 30mins

Ingredients:

2 cups plain yogurt

1 cucumber, cut lengthwise

1 ¼ tbsp. salt

1 clove garlic, crushed

¼ tbsp. dill

2 tbsp. extra-virgin olive oil

1 ½ tbsp. lemon juice

1 tbsp. oregano

1 ⅓ lb. chicken breasts, cubed

4 whole-wheat pitas

1 tbsp. capers

1 red onion, cut into wedges

2 tomatoes, cut into wedges

⅓ cup black olives, pitted

Directions:

Put the yogurt in a strainer lined with cheesecloth and set it over a bowl to drain some liquid. In a colander, add the cucumber with 1 tbsp. of salt; let sit for around 15 minutes.

Squeeze the cucumber and finely chop it. Put it in a bowl and add the yogurt, garlic, 1/8 tbsp. of pepper, and dill.

Warm the grill. Combine the oil, lemon juice, oregano, 1/4 tbsp. of salt, and 1/4 tbsp. of pepper.

Toss the chicken cubes in the oil blend and thread them onto skewers. Grill the chicken over high heat, turning once until done, about 10 to 12 minutes.

Grill the pitas for 1 minute per side, cut them in half. Put them on serving dishes and top them with the onion, tomatoes, and chicken skewers.

Serve with the yogurt sauce and olives on the side.

NUTRITION FACTS: CALORIES 356KCAL FAT 9 G CARBOHYDRATE 25 G PROTEIN 14 G

SALMON FRITTERS

 2   🕐 30 mins

Ingredients:

6 oz. salmon, canned
1 tbsp. flour
1 garlic clove, crushed
½ red onion, finely chopped
2 eggs
2 tsp. olive oil
Salt and pepper to taste
2 cups arugula

Directions:

Separate egg whites from yolks and beat them until very stiff. In a separate bowl, mix salmon, flour, salt, pepper, onion, garlic, and yolks.

Add egg whites and mix slowly. Heat a pan on medium-high. Add 1 tsp. oil and, when hot, form salmon fritters with a spoon.

Cook until brown (around 4 minutes per side) and serve with arugula salad seasoned with salt, pepper, and 1 tsp. olive oil.

NUTRITION FACTS: CALORIES 320KCAL FAT 7 G CARBOHYDRATE 18 G PROTEIN 27 G

SEARED TUNA IN SOY SAUCE AND BLACK PEPPER 1   🕐 35 mins

Ingredients:

5 ounces tuna, 1-inch thick
1 red onion, chopped
2 tbsp. soy sauce
¼ tsp. ground black pepper
½ tbsp. grated ginger
1 tsp. sesame seeds
2 tsp. extra-virgin olive oil
2 cups baby spinach
1 tbsp. orange juice

Directions:

Marinate tuna with 1 tbsp. soy sauce, oil, and black pepper for 30 minutes. Place a skillet over high heat and, when very hot, add tuna and quickly cook 1 minute per side.

Cut the tuna into slices, dress them with 1 tbsp. soy sauce mixed with grated ginger. Add green onion and sesame seeds on top.

Serve with a baby spinach salad dressed with 1 tsp olive oil, salt, pepper, and orange juice.

NUTRITION FACTS: CALORIES 154KCAL FAT 4.1 G CARBOHYDRATE 3 G PROTEIN 15 G

SERRANO HAM & ARUGULA

 2 10 mins

Ingredients:
6 oz. Serrano ham
4 oz. arugula leaves
2 tbsp. olive oil
1 tbsp. orange juice

Directions:
Pour the oil and juice into a bowl and toss the arugula in the mixture. Place the arugula mixture on plates and top off with the ham.

NUTRITION FACTS: CALORIES 220KCAL FAT 7 G CARBOHYDRATE 7 G PROTEIN 33.5 G

SESAME TUNA WITH ARTICHOKE HEARTS

 2 35 mins

Ingredients:
8 oz. tuna steaks
2 tbsp. white sesame
2 tbsp. black sesame
1 tsp. sesame oil
2 artichokes
2 tsp. extra-virgin olive oil
½ lemon, juiced
1 garlic clove
1 handful parsley

Directions:
Discard the outer leaves, and then slice artichokes very fine. Heat a pan with olive oil, add garlic and cook for a couple of minutes, then remove the clove. Add artichokes, lemon, salt, and pepper. Cook 5-10 minutes until tender. Set aside.

Mix sesame seeds and press them on tuna until it is completely covered.

Heat a pan and add sesame oil. When the oil is very hot, cook tuna for 1-2 minutes per side.

Serve tuna alongside artichokes.

NUTRITION FACTS: CALORIES 353KCAL FAT 4.8 G CARBOHYDRATE 28.1 G PROTEIN 28.3 G

MINCE STUFFED PEPPERS

🍴 4   🕐 75 mins

Ingredients:
4 oz. lean mince
¼ cup brown rice, cooked
2 yellow bell peppers
2 red bell peppers
1 tbsp. parmesan
2 tbsp. breadcrumbs
3 oz. mozzarella
1 egg
¼ cup walnuts, chopped
2 cups arugula
2 tsp. extra-virgin olive oil
A few drops of lemon juice

Directions:
Preheat oven to 350 degrees F.

In a bowl, mix the mince, parmesan, brown rice, egg, and mozzarella. Mix well and set aside.

Cut peppers lengthwise, remove the seeds, fill them with the mince mix, and put them on a baking tray. Distribute breadcrumbs on top and lightly spray with cooking spray to have a crunchy top without adding calories to the recipe.

Cook for 50-60 minutes until peppers are soft. Let cool for a few minutes.

Serve stuffed peppers with an arugula salad dressed with olive oil, salt, and a few lemon drops.

NUTRITION FACTS: CALORIES 375KCAL FAT 8.2 G CARBOHYDRATE 24.7 G PROTEIN 15.3 G

MOROCCAN SPICED EGGS

🍴 2   🕐 55 mins

Ingredients:
1 tsp. extra-virgin olive oil
1 scallion, finely chopped
1 red bell pepper, finely chopped
1 garlic clove, finely chopped
1 zucchini, finely chopped
1 tbsp. tomato paste
½ tsp. mild curry
¼ tsp. ground cinnamon
¼ tsp. ground cumin
½ tsp. salt
1 can tomatoes
1 can chickpeas, drained
1/3 oz. parsley
4 eggs

Directions:
Heat the oil in a pan; include the scallion and red bell pepper and fry on low heat for 5 minutes. Add garlic and zucchini and cook for 2 minutes. Add tomato paste, spices, and salt and stir well.

Add tomatoes and chickpeas and bring to medium heat. Put a lid on and simmer for 30 minutes until thicker. Remove from heat and add chopped parsley. Preheat the grill to 350°F.

Spread the tomato sauce into a cooking tray and crack the eggs in the middle. Put the tray under the grill for 10 minutes and serve.

NUTRITION FACTS: CALORIES 316KCAL FAT 5.2 G CARBOHYDRATE 13.1 G PROTEIN 7 G

MISO CARAMELIZED TOFU

🍳 2   🕐 45 mins

Ingredients:

1 tbsp. mirin
¾ oz. miso paste
10 oz. firm tofu
2 oz. celery, trimmed
2 oz. red onion
4 ¼ oz. zucchini
1 garlic clove, finely chopped
1 tsp. fresh ginger, finely chopped
5 oz. kale, chopped
2 tsp. sesame seeds
1 ¼ oz. buckwheat
1 tsp. ground turmeric
2 tsp. extra-virgin olive oil
1 tsp. tamari (or soy sauce)

Preheat your oven to 400°F. Cover a tray with parchment paper. Combine the mirin and miso. Dice the tofu and let it marinate in the mirin-miso mixture. Chop the vegetables (except for the kale) at a diagonal angle to produce long slices.

Using a steamer, cook the kale for 5 minutes and set aside. Disperse the tofu across the lined tray and garnish with sesame seeds. Roast for 20 minutes, or until caramelized. Rinse the buckwheat using running water and a sieve.

Add to a pan of boiling water with turmeric and cook the buckwheat according to the packet instructions.

Heat the oil in a skillet over high heat. Toss in the vegetables, herbs, and spices, then fry for 2 to 3 minutes. Reduce to medium heat and fry for another 5 minutes or until cooked but still crunchy.

Directions:

NUTRITION FACTS: CALORIES 101KCAL   FAT 4.7 G   CARBOHYDRATE 12.4 G   PROTEIN 4.2 G

CHIPOTLE CITRUS-GLAZED TURKEY TENDERLOINS

🍳 4　　🕐 25 mins

Ingredients:

4 5 oz. turkey breast tenderloins
¼ tsp. salt
¼ tsp. pepper
1 tbsp. extra-virgin olive oil
1 garlic clove, crushed
¾ cup orange juice
¼ cup lime juice
1 tsp. agave syrup
2 tsp. minced chipotle peppers
2 tbsp. parsley, chopped

Directions:

Season turkey with salt and pepper. Cook it in a skillet with ½ tbsp. oil over high heat.

Meanwhile, in a bowl, whisk the orange juice, lime juice, agave, ½ tbsp. oil, and chipotle.

Add the sauce to the skillet. Reduce heat and simmer for 14 to 16 minutes. Transfer turkey to a cutting board; let rest for 5 minutes.

Simmer glaze until thickened, about 3 minutes. Slice the turkey, top with parsley, and serve with glaze.

NUTRITION FACTS: CALORIES 294KCAL FAT 6 G CARBOHYDRATE 9 G PROTEIN 30 G

COCONUT SHRIMP

🍳 2　　🕐 30 mins

Ingredients:

½ cup buckwheat flour
1 ½ tbsp. pepper
2 eggs
⅔ cup dried coconut, shredded
⅓ cup panko (Japanese-style breadcrumbs)
12 oz. deveined shrimp, tail-on
½ tbsp. salt
¼ cup agave syrup
¼ cup lime juice
2 tbsp. parsley, chopped

Directions:

Mix flour and pepper in a shallow dish. Gently beat eggs in another dish and mix coconut and panko in a third one.

Holding each shrimp by the tail, dip them in flour, paing attention to not cover the tail; shake off excess. Dunk in egg, allowing any excess to trickle off.

Dip in coconut blend and coat well. Put the shrimp in oven, and cook at 400°F until golden, 5 to 6 minutes, turning them over halfway through cooking. season with 1/4 tbsp. of the salt.

While shrimp cook, whisk together nectar, lime juice, and serrano chile in a bowl. Sprinkle shrimp with parsley. Serve with sauce.

NUTRITION FACTS: CALORIES 250KCAL FAT 6 G CARBOHYDRATE 20 G PROTEIN 15 G

GARLIC CHICKEN BURGERS

 2   20 mins

Ingredients:
10 oz. chicken mince
¼ red onion, finely chopped
1 clove garlic, crushed
1 handful of parsley, finely chopped
1 cup arugula
½ orange, chopped
1 cup cherry tomatoes
3 tsp extra-virgin olive oil

Directions:
Put chicken mince, onion, garlic, parsley, salt, and pepper to taste in a bowl and mix well.

Form 2 patties and let rest 5 minutes. Heat a pan with olive oil, and when very hot, cook 3 minutes per side.

Put the arugula on two plates; add cherry tomatoes and orange, dress with salt and the remaining olive oil. Put the patties on top and serve.

These patties are delicious also when grilled. If you opt for grilling, just brush them with a bit of extra-virgin olive oil right before cooking.

NUTRITION FACTS: CALORIES 253KCAL FAT 4.8 G CARBOHYDRATE 8.1 G PROTEIN 28.3 G

LIME-PARSLEY COD

 4   15 mins

Ingredients:
4 6-oz. cod fillets
½ tsp. salt
¼ tsp. pepper
3 tbsp. extra-virgin olive oil
1 cup arugula
2 tbsp. parsley, chopped
1 tbsp. lime juice
1 tsp. lime zest

Directions:
Preheat oven to 375°F. Mix the salt, pepper, 2 tsp. olive oil, lime juice, and zest in a bowl and whisk.

Put the cod fillets on a baking dish greased with cooking spray or one drop of extra virgin olive oil.

Pour the sauce over the fish and cook 6 to 8 minutes until done. Top with parsley.

Serve with a simple side of arugula seasoned with salt, pepper, and 1 tbsp. olive oil.

NUTRITION FACTS: CALORIES 245KCAL FAT 3 G CARBOHYDRATE 5 G PROTEIN 28 G

HERBS AND CHEESE BURGERS

🍳 4   🕐 *25 mins*

Ingredients:

2 green onions, chopped
½ red onion, chopped
2 tbsp. parsley, chopped
4 tbsp. Dijon mustard
3 tbsp. breadcrumbs
½ tbsp. salt
½ tbsp. rosemary
¼ tbsp. sage
1 lb. lean mincemeat
2 oz. cheddar, shredded
4 buckwheat burger buns

Directions:

Preheat oven to 375°F. In a bowl, mix green onions, parsley, and 2 tbsp. mustard. In another bowl, mix breadcrumbs, red onion, sage, rosemary, and remaining 2 tbsp. mustard.

Add mincemeat and mix well using a fork or the hands. Shape into 8 patties. T

ake one patty, put a tsp. of cheddar, and a tsp. of green onion blend.

Top with another patty, and gently squeeze edges together to seal them well.

Place burgers in a baking dish and cook 6 to 8 minutes.

Serve burgers with buns, topped with arugula.

NUTRITION FACTS: CALORIES 369KCAL FAT 14 G CARBOHYDRATE 29 G PROTEIN 29 G

ITALIAN-STYLE MEATBALLS

🍳 4   🕐 45 mins

Ingredients:

2 tbsp. extra-virgin olive oil
1 medium shallot
3 cloves garlic, crushed
2-inch celery, finely diced
¼ cup buckwheat breadcrumb
2 tbsp. milk
10 oz. lean mincemeat
10 oz. turkey mincemeat
1 egg
¼ cup parsley, chopped
1 tbsp. rosemary
1 tbsp. thyme
1 tbsp. Dijon mustard

Directions:

Preheat Oven to 400°F.

Heat oil in a skillet over medium-high. Add shallot and cook until soft, about 2 minutes. Add garlic and cook 1 minute. Remove from heat. In a bowl, mix breadcrumb and milk. Add shallot and garlic, mincemeat, egg, parsley, rosemary, thyme, mustard, and salt. Mix.

Gently shape blend into small balls and put them on a tray in a single layer. Cook at 400°F until caramelized and cooked through, about 15 to 18 minutes.

Serve hot.

NUTRITION FACTS: CALORIES 322KCAL FAT 8 G CARBOHYDRATE 5 G PROTEIN 17 G

KALE OMELETTE

 1   🕙 10 mins

Ingredients:
2 eggs
1 small clove garlic
2 handfuls kale
1 oz. goat cheese
¼ cup sliced onion
2 teaspoons extra virgin olive oil

Directions:
Mince the garlic and finely shred the kale. Break the eggs into a bowl, add a pinch of salt. Beat until well combined.

Place a pan over medium heat. Add 1 teaspoon of olive oil, add the onion and kale, cook for approx. 5 minutes, or until the onion has softened and the kale is wilted.

Add the garlic and cook for another 2 minutes.

Add 1 teaspoon of olive oil into the egg mixture, mix and add into the pan. Use your spatula to move the cooked egg toward the center and move the pan so that the uncooked egg mixture goes towards the edges.

Add the cheese into the pan just before the egg is fully cooked, then leave for 1 minute.

Serve immediately.

NUTRITION FACTS: CALORIES 219KCAL FAT 8 G CARBOHYDRATE 7.7 G PROTEIN 12 G

LEMON-FENNEL SPICY COD

 4 15 mins

Ingredients:
1 tbsp. ground coriander
3 tbsp. extra-virgin olive oil
2 garlic cloves, crushed
4 6-ounce cod fillets
2 cups fennel, finely sliced
1/4 cup red onion, chopped
2 tbsp. lemon juice
1 tbsp. parsley, chopped
1 tbsp. thyme leaves, chopped

Directions:
Combine coriander, 2 tbsp. oil, garlic, salt, and pepper to taste in a bowl. Rub garlic blend over the cod fillets.

Warm a skillet over medium-high heat. Add the cod and cook for 5 to 6 minutes on each side. In the meantime, add fennel, onion, lemon juice, 1 tbsp. oil, thyme, and parsley in a bowl, tossing to cover.

Serve a plate of fennel salad with a cod fillet on top.

NUTRITION FACTS: CALORIES 259KCAL FAT 9.7 G CARBOHYDRATE 5.3 G PROTEIN 18 G

RED ONION FRITTATA WITH GRILLED ZUCCHINI

 2 35 mins

Ingredients:
1 ½ cups red onion, finely sliced
3 eggs
3 oz. cheddar cheese
2 tbsp. milk
2 zucchini
2 tbsp. oil
1 clove garlic, crushed
1 tsp. white vinegar
Salt and pepper to taste

Directions:
Heat the oven to 350°F. Cut the zucchini into thin slices, grill them, and set them aside.

Add 3 eggs, shredded cheddar cheese, milk, salt, and pepper. Whisk well and pour in a silicone baking tray and cook 25-30 minutes in the oven. Mix garlic, oil, salt, pepper, and vinegar and pour the dressing on the zucchini. Serve the frittata alongside the zucchini.

NUTRITION FACTS: CALORIES 229KCAL FAT 7.8 G CARBOHYDRATE 8.1 G PROTEIN 21.3 G

MINCE STUFFED EGGPLANTS

 6   🕐 50 mins

Ingredients:

8 oz. lean mincemeat
6 large eggplants
1 egg
3 tbsp. dry red wine
½ cup cheddar, grated
Salt and pepper, to taste
1 red onion
2 tsp. olive oil
2 tbsp. tomato sauce
2 tbsp. parsley

Directions:

Preheat oven to 350°F. Meanwhile, slice eggplants in half and scoop out the center part, leaving ½" of meat. Place eggplants in a microwavable dish with about ½" of water in the bottom.

Microwave on high for 4 minutes. In a saucepan, fry mince with onion for 5 minutes. Add wine and let evaporate. Add tomato sauce, salt, pepper, eggplant meat, and cook for 20 minutes

Combine mince sauce, cheese, egg, parsley, salt, and pepper in a large bowl and mix well. Pack firmly into eggplants.

Return eggplants to the dish you first microwaved them in and bake for 25 to 30 minutes, or until lightly browned on top.

NUTRITION FACTS: CALORIES 350KCAL FAT 10 G CARBOHYDRATE 22 G PROTEIN 17 G

MUSTARD SALMON WITH BABY CARROTS

🍲 2   🕐 50 mins

Ingredients:
12 oz. salmon fillet
2 tbsp. mustard
1 tbsp. white vinegar
1 tsp parsley, finely chopped
2 cups baby carrots
4 oz. buckwheat
2 tsp. extra virgin olive oil
Salt and pepper to taste

Directions:
Heat the oven to 400°F.
Boil the buckwheat in salted water for 25 minutes then drain. Dress with 1 tsp olive oil. Set aside.
Put the salmon over aluminum foil.
Mix mustard and vinegar in a small bowl and brush the mixture over the salmon, close the foil in a packet. Cook in the oven 35minutes.
While the salmon is cooking, steam baby carrots for 6 minutes then put them in a pan on medium heat with 1tsp. olive oil, salt and pepper until light brown.
Serve the salmon with baby carrots and buckwheat on the side.

NUTRITION FACTS: CALORIES 357KCAL FAT 9.1 G CARBOHYDRATE 8 G PROTEIN 26 G

ROASTED SALMON WITH FENNEL SALAD

🍲 4   🕐 25mins

Ingredients:
2 tbsp. parsley
1 tbsp. thyme
1 tbsp. genuine salt,
4 6-oz. skinless salmon fillets
2 tbsp. extra-virgin olive oil
4 cups fennel, finely sliced
2/3 cup low-fat Greek yogurt
1 garlic clove, crushed
2 tbsp. orange juice
1 tbsp. lemon juice
2 tbsp. dill
½ tsp. turmeric

Directions:
Preheat oven to 200°F.
Mix parsley, thyme, and 1/2 tbsp. of the salt in a little bowl. Brush salmon with oil; sprinkle equally with herb blend.
Put salmon fillets in an oven-proof skillet, and cook at 350°F until desired doneness level, 10 minutes.
While salmon cooks, toss together fennel, yogurt, garlic, squeezed orange, lemon juice, dill, and 1/2 tbsp. salt in a medium bowl. Serve salmon ts over the fennel plate of mixed greens.

NUTRITION FACTS: CALORIES 364KCAL FAT 9 G CARBOHYDRATE 9 G PROTEIN 27 G

SALMON FRITTERS

 2   🕐 20 mins

Ingredients:
6 oz. salmon, canned
1 tbsp. flour
1 clove garlic, crushed
½ red onion, finely chopped
2 eggs
2 tsp. olive oil
Salt and pepper to taste
2 cups arugula

Directions:
Separate egg whites from yolks and beat them until very stiff. In a separate bowl, mix salmon, flour, salt, pepper, onion, garlic, and yolks.

Add egg whites and mix slowly. Heat a pan on medium-high. Add 1 tsp. oil and, when hot, form salmon fritters with a spoon.

Cook until brown (around 4 minutes per side) and serve with arugula salad seasoned with salt, pepper, and 1 tsp. olive oil.

NUTRITION FACTS: CALORIES 320KCAL FAT 7 G CARBOHYDRATE 18 G PROTEIN 27 G

SPICY CHICKEN BREASTS

 8   🕐 25 mins + 1h

Ingredients:
2 cups buttermilk
2 tbsp. Dijon mustard
1 pinch of salt
2 tbsp. hot pepper sauce
1-1/2 tbsp. garlic powder
8 chicken breast, skinless
2 cups buckwheat breadcrumbs
2 tbsp. extra-virgin olive oil
1/2 tbsp. paprika
1/4 tbsp. dried oregano
1/4 tbsp. dried parsley
2 tsp. capers, finely chopped

Directions:
Preheat oven to 375°F. Marinate the chicken in buttermilk with mustard and hot sauce for at least 1 hour.

Drain the chicken. Mix garlic, salt, paprika, oregano, parsley, and capers with breadcrumbs and coat the chicken.

Put the chicken on a tray in a single layer. Cook for 18 to 20 minutes, turning one time halfway.

Serve hot.

NUTRITION FACTS: CALORIES 352KCAL FAT 9 G CARBOHYDRATE 11 G PROTEIN 24 G

SHRIMP SPRING ROLLS

4   35 mins

Ingredients:

1 tbsp. sesame oil
1 tbsp. extra-virgin olive oil
½ cup cabbage, shredded
½ cup carrots
½ red pepper
½ red onion
4 oz. shrimp, finely chopped
½ cup snow peas
1/4 cup parsley, chopped
1 tbsp. lime juice
2 tbsp. fish sauce
16 (8-inch-square) phyllo batter sheets

Directions:

Cut carrots into matchsticks and finely chop snow peas, red pepper, and onion. Warm oil in a skillet over high heat.

Add cabbage, carrots, onion, snow peas, and red pepper; cook for 3 minutes. Let cool for 5 minutes. Put cabbage blend, shrimp, parsley, lime juice, fish sauce; toss to combine. Preheat the oven to 400°F.

Put one phyllo sheet on a work surface, lightly damp it with one drop of water, and cover with a second sheet.

Put 1/8 of the filling on one side, then roll the sheets to form a spring roll. Cook the spring rolls until golden, 6 to 7 minutes, turning them after 4 minutes.

NUTRITION FACTS: CALORIES 280KCAL FAT 9 G CARBOHYDRATE 19 G PROTEIN 7 G

SOUTHERN STYLE CATFISH WITH GREEN BEANS

 2   🕐 35 mins

Ingredients:
2 6-oz. catfish fillets
¼ cup flour
1 egg
½ cup buckwheat breadcrumbs
¼ tbsp. pepper
12 oz. green beans
2 tbsp. mayonnaise
1 ½ tbsp. dill
¾ tbsp. dill pickle relish
½ tsp. red wine vinegar
1 tsp agave syrup
1 tbsp. extra-virgin olive oil

Directions:
Steam green beans for 20 minutes. In the meantime prepare flour, egg, and breadcrumbs on three different plates.

Briefly whisk the egg; then first, coat catfish in flour, shaking excess. Then dip one piece of fish at a time in the egg and cover with breadcrumbs on all sides.

Place fish on a baking tray, drizzle olive oil on top, and cook at 400°F for 10 to 12 minutes, until crispy.

While the fish is cooking, whisk mayonnaise, dill, relish, vinegar, and agave in a bowl to form a sauce.

Serve the catfish and green beans with sauce.

NUTRITION FACTS: CALORIES 316KCAL FAT 8 G CARBOHYDRATE 11 G PROTEIN 33 G

TURMERIC COUS COUS WITH EDAMAME BEANS

🍲 2   🕐 25 mins

Ingredients:

½ yellow pepper, cubed
½ red pepper, cubed
1 tbsp. turmeric
½ cup red onion, finely sliced
¼ cup cherry tomatoes, chopped
2 tbsp. parsley, finely chopped
5 oz. couscous
2 tsp. extra virgin olive oil
½ eggplant
1 ½ cup edamame beans

Directions:

Steam edamame for 5 minutes and set aside. Add 6 oz. salted boiling water to couscous and let rest until it absorbs the water.

In the meantime, heat a pan on medium-high heat. Add oil, eggplant, peppers, onion, tomatoes, turmeric, salt, and pepper.

Cook for 5 minutes on high heat. Add the couscous and edamame.

Garnish with fresh parsley and serve.

NUTRITION FACTS: CALORIES 342KCAL FAT 5 G CARBOHYDRATE 15 G PROTEIN 32 G

TURMERIC TURKEY BREAST WITH CAULIFLOWER RICE

🍲 2   🕐 25 mins

Ingredients:

2 cups cauliflower, grated
8 oz. turkey breast, cut into slices
2 tsp. ground turmeric
1/2 pepper, chopped
1/2 red onion, sliced
2 tsp. extra virgin olive oil
1 large tomato
1 clove garlic, crushed
1 cup milk, skimmed
2 tsp. buckwheat flour
1 oz. parsley, finely chopped

Directions:

Coat turkey slices with flour. Heat a pan on medium-high with half the oil, and when hot, add the turkey.

Let the meat color on all sides, then add milk, salt, pepper, 1 tsp. turmeric. Cook 10 minutes until the turkey is soft, and the sauce has become creamy.

Warm another pan with the remaining oil over medium heat.. Add pepper, onion, and tomato, 1 tsp. turmeric, and let cook 3 minutes. Add the cauliflower and cook another 2 minutes. Add salt and pepper to taste. Let rest 2 minutes.

Serve the turkey with the cauliflower rice.

NUTRITION FACTS: CALORIES 187KCAL FAT 2.9 G CARBOHYDRATE 10.6 G PROTEIN 12.1 G

ASIAN NOODLE SOUP

2   30 mins

Ingredients:

2 cups vegetable broth
1 egg
2 cups of spinach
1 cup zucchini, chopped
6 oz. shrimp
6 oz. chicken breast
2 oz. bean sprouts
1 stalk celery, chopped
1 packet of Konjak noodles
1 tbsp. soy sauce
1 tbsp. fish sauce
1 handful fresh parsley
1-inch ginger, peel and chopped

Directions:

Boil the egg for 7 minutes, then drain it and cool it under running water.

Cook the shrimp and chicken in the broth with the spices and chopped vegetables for 15 minutes.

Wash the noodles under running water, add them to the soup and let them warm for 2 minutes.

Put the soup in a bowl, top with half egg, bean sprouts, and parsley, and serve.

NUTRITION FACTS: CALORIES 264KCAL FAT 6 G CARBOHYDRATE 19 G PROTEIN 8 G

ASPARAGUS CREAM SOUP

🍲 2   🕐 25 mins

Ingredients:
2 cups asparagus
3 cups vegetable broth
2 tbsp. extra-virgin olive oil
2 tbsp. flour
1 egg yolk
2 tbsp. cream
1 handful parsley, chopped

Directions:
Chop the asparagus. Boil the asparagus for 15 minutes in salted water. Drain them and add them back to the pot. In a pan, heat 1 tbsp. extra-virgin olive oil, add the flour, and ½ cup broth.

Whisk in the egg yolks and the cream. Add it to the pot with asparagus and the remaining broth, add the parsley and blend with a hand blender for 2 to 3 minutes until very smooth.

Divide into 2 plates, add the remaining extra-virgin olive oil on top and serve.

NUTRITION FACTS: CALORIES 253KCAL FAT 5 G CARBOHYDRATE 19 G PROTEIN 12 G

BROCCOLI AND WALNUT SOUP

 6   🕐 40 mins

Ingredients:
2 cups broccoli
½ cup walnuts
4 cups vegetable stock
2 tbsp. cream
Fresh nutmeg

Directions:
Cut the broccoli into florets, and then boil them in vegetable stock for 8 to 10 minutes.

Blend the walnuts in a blender, then add the broccoli and broth and blend again for 2 to 3 minutes. Season it with salt and pepper to taste, nutmeg and quickly blend again.

Serve.

NUTRITION FACTS: CALORIES 264KCAL FAT 8 G CARBOHYDRATE 17 G PROTEIN 9 G

BROCCOLI, CHEDDAR AND CHICKEN SOUP

 4 39 mins

Ingredients:
3 tbsp. extra-virgin olive oil
1 cup red onion, diced
1 cup celery, diced
½ cup flour
1 tsp. mustard
¼ tsp. salt
¼ tsp. ground pepper
4 cups chicken stock
1 cup milk
3 cups broccoli
2 cups potatoes, diced
1 lb. chicken breast, diced
1 cup cheddar, shredded

Directions:
Heat oil in a pan over medium heat. Add onion and celery, and cook 5 minutes until the onion becomes transparent.

Sprinkle flour, mustard, salt, and pepper over the vegetables and cook, for 2 minutes. Add the stock and milk; bring to a boil and add the chicken, broccoli, and potatoes.

Cook until the potatoes are soft and the chicken is done, about 12 to 14 minutes.

Add the cheddar, let melt for 2 minutes and serve.

NUTRITION FACTS: CALORIES 3144CAL   FAT 3 G   CARBOHYDRATE 19 G   PROTEIN 21 G

CAULIFLOWER SOUP

 4 30 mins

Ingredients:
2 cups cauliflower
3 oz. bacon
1 tsp. extra-virgin olive oil
2 tbsp. parmesan, grated
3 cups vegetable broth
1 pinch nutmeg
1 tbsp. capers

Directions:
Stew the cauliflower with a little water for 18 minutes.

Drain it, then blend it with warm broth until creamy. Season with nutmeg, capers., salt, and pepper to taste.

Fry the bacon in a pan. Serve the soup in a bowl, garnished with bacon, parmesan, and olive oil on top.

NUTRITION FACTS: CALORIES 289KCAL   FAT 8 G   CARBOHYDRATE 13 G   PROTEIN 18 G

CAULIFLOWER AND MUSHROOM SOUP

 6   ◷ 55 mins

Ingredients:

35 oz. chicken fillet
1 red onion
1 tbsp. olive oil
2 garlic cloves, crushed
6 sun-dried tomatoes
2 cups mushrooms, sliced
2 cups cauliflower
1 zucchini, chopped
½ cup green beans
1 cup kale, chopped
2 tbsp. red wine vinegar
1 bay leaf
1 handful parsley

Directions:

Boil the chicken in salted water with half onion and the bay leaf. Cook on low heat for 50 minutes, then remove the meat and shred it with a fork. Set aside.

While the chicken is cooking, heat the oil in a skillet, add the remaining half onion, finely chopped, garlic, sun-dried tomatoes, and mushrooms.

Add the broth, cauliflower, zucchini, and green beans and let it simmer for 15 minutes. Then add the leafy vegetables cut in pieces and let them cook for another 10 minutes.

Serve in bowls, adding the shredded chicken and parsley on top.

NUTRITION FACTS: CALORIES 236KCAL FAT 3 G CARBOHYDRATE 17 G PROTEIN 11 G

PEAR AND CELERY SOUP

6   35 mins

Ingredients:
5 cups finely chopped celery
4 onions, chopped
¼ cup chives
½ tsp. dried thyme
½ tsp. salt
¼ tsp. pepper
6 cups vegetable stock
3 ripe pears, peeled, cored, and chopped
½ cup 10% cream

Directions:
Heat extra-virgin olive oil in a saucepan.

Cook celery, onions, chives, thyme, salt, and pepper, covered and occasionally stirring, for about 10 minutes.

Pour in the stock and bring to boil. Reduce heat and simmer until the celery is tender, about 10 minutes.

Add pears; cook for 5 minutes or until pears are tender. Purée in a blender.

Return to saucepan; pour in cream and heat through without boiling.

Serve hot.

NUTRITION FACTS: CALORIES 116KCAL FAT 4 G CARBOHYDRATE 13 G PROTEIN 7 G

PUMPKIN SOUP WITH PUMPKIN SEEDS AND GINGER

🍲 4   🕐 25 mins

Ingredients:
3 cups pumpkin, chopped
2 carrots
1 shallot
1 red onion
1 ¼ in. ginger
3 cups water
2 tbsp. pumpkin seeds
1 tbsp. extra-virgin olive oil

Directions:
Peel and dice the carrots. Peel the shallot and finely chop it Sauté the shallot in a saucepan with oil.

Add the squash and carrots and sauté them for 5 minutes. Pour boiling water and simmer over medium heat for 15 minutes.

Peel and grate the ginger. Add it to the soup, then blend it with a hand blender until smooth.

Season the soup with lime juice, salt, and pepper to taste. Top with pumpkin seeds and serve.

NUTRITION FACTS: CALORIES 127KCAL   FAT 3 G   CARBOHYDRATE 15 G   PROTEIN 4 G

ROASTED CAULIFLOWER AND POTATO CURRY SOUP

🍲 4   🕐 40 mins

Ingredients:

2 tsp. ground cumin
½ tsp. ground cinnamon
1 ½ tsp. turmeric
⅛ tsp. cayenne pepper
1 cauliflower, chopped into florets
2 tbsp. extra-virgin olive oil
1 red onion
1 cup carrot, chopped
3 cloves garlic, crushed
1 ½ tsp. ginger, grated
14 oz. tomato sauce
4 cups vegetable stock
1 potato, diced
1 sweet potato, diced
1 handful parsley, chopped

Directions:

Preheat the oven to 400°F. Mix parsley, cumin, cinnamon, turmeric, salt, pepper, and cayenne in a bowl.

Toss cauliflower with 1 tbsp. oil in a bowl, add the spices mix, and toss again to cover. Transfer the cauliflower to a baking dish and cook it in the oven until caramelized, about 15 to 20 minutes.

In the meantime, heat 1 tbsp.oil in a pot over medium-high heat. Add onion and carrot and cook for 5 minutes until they are both soft. Lower the heat, and add garlic, and ginger.

Cook for 1 minute, then add the tomato sauce, stock, potato, and sweet potato. Bring to a boil and simmer for 20 minutes.

Mix in coconut milk and the cooked cauliflower and warm through. Trim with parsley and serve.

NUTRITION FACTS: CALORIES 120KCAL   FAT 3 G   CARBOHYDRATE 10 G   PROTEIN 8 G

MEDITERRANEAN CHICKPEA SOUP

 6   2h + 5mins

Ingredients:

1 ½ cups dried chickpeas, soaked overnight
2 lbs. turkey breast
1 red onion, finely chopped
I celery stalk, chopped
15 oz. tomatoes, diced
2 tbsp. tomato paste
4 cloves garlic
2 tsp. turmeric
I tsp. sage
I tsp. marjoram
14 oz. artichoke hearts
2 tbsp. extra-virgin olive oil
¼ cup parsley, chopped

Directions:

Drain chickpeas and put them in a pot. Add 6 cups of water, onion, tomatoes, tomato paste, garlic, turmeric. Bring to a boil.

Add the turkey and bring back to a boil, lower the heat, and cook, covered, for 75 minutes. Season with salt to taste, add artichokes, and cook for another 15 minutes.

The turkey should now be cooked. If so, remove it from the pot and set aside, if not keep cooking with the soup until done.

Chickpeas cook in about 2 hours. Shred the turkey with a fork and mix it back into the soup.

Sprinkle chopped parsley on top and serve.

NUTRITION FACTS: CALORIES 280KCAL FAT 3 G CARBOHYDRATE 26 G PROTEIN 23 G

SQUASH AND CORN SOUP

 4   50 mins

Ingredients:

3 tbsp. extra-virgin olive oil
1 cup red onion, diced
1 cup celery, diced
½ cup flour
1 ½ tsp. dried marjoram
4 cups vegetable broth
1 cup milk
3 cups summer squash, diced
2 cups red potatoes, diced
1 cup corn
¾ cup ham, diced

Directions:

Sautè the celery and onion in a skillet with oil for minutes until soft. Add flour and marjoram, season with salt and pepper to taste, and cook, mixing, for 2 minutes.

Add the broth and milk; bring to a boil, and squash, potatoes, and corn.

Stew, until the potatoes are tender, about 14 minutes.

Add ham, warm through and serve.

NUTRITION FACTS: CALORIES 285KCAL FAT 7 G CARBOHYDRATE 16 G PROTEIN 18 G

SALADS

CELERY AND RAISINS SNACK SALAD

 4   10 mins

Ingredients:
½ cup raisins
4 cups celery, sliced
¼ cup parsley, chopped
½ cup walnuts, chopped
Juice of ½ lemon
2 tbsp. extra virgin olive oil
Salt and black pepper to the taste

Directions:
   In a salad bowl, mix celery with raisins, walnuts, parsley, lemon juice, oil, and black pepper, toss, divide into small cups and serve as a snack.

NUTRITION FACTS: CALORIES 120KCAL FAT 3 G CARBOHYDRATE 6 G PROTEIN 5 G

DIJON CELERY SALAD

 4   🕐 10 mins

Ingredients:
2 tsp. honey
½ lemon, juiced
1 tbsp. Dijon mustard
2 tsp. extra virgin olive oil
Black pepper to taste
2 apples, cored, peeled, and cubed
1 bunch celery roughly chopped
¾ cup walnuts, chopped

Directions:
In a salad bowl, mix celery and its leaves with apple pieces and walnuts.

Add black pepper, lemon juice, mustard, honey, and olive oil.

Whisk well, add to the salad, toss, and serve.

NUTRITION FACTS: CALORIES 125KCAL FAT 2 G CARBOHYDRATE 7 G PROTEIN 7 G

EASY SHRIMP SALAD

 2   5 mins

Ingredients:
2 cups red endive, finely sliced
1 cup cherry tomatoes, halved
1 tsp. of extra virgin olive oil
1 tbsp. parsley, chopped
3 oz. celery, sliced
6 walnuts, chopped
2 oz. red onion-sliced
1 cup yellow pepper, cubed
½ lemon, juiced
6 oz. steamed shrimp

Directions:
Put red endive on a large plate. Evenly distribute finely sliced onion on top, yellow pepper, cherry tomatoes, walnuts, celery, parsley, and shrimp.

Mix oil and lemon juice, with a pinch of salt and pepper, and distribute the dressing on top.

NUTRITION FACTS: CALORIES 232KCAL FAT 4.8 G CARBOHYDRATE 13 G PROTEIN 18 G

SNACKS

AVOCADO FRIES

 4   🕐 20 mins

Ingredients:
½ cup flour
1 ½ tbsp. pepper
2 eggs
½ cup panko (Japanese-style breadcrumbs)
2 avocados, chopped into 8 wedges each
¼ tbsp salt
2 tbsp. ketchup
2 tbsp. mayonnaise
1 tbsp. apple juice vinegar
1 tbsp. Sriracha sauce
1 tbsp. turmeric

Directions:
Mix flour, a pinch of salt, and pepper in a shallow dish. Delicately beat eggs and water in another dish and panko in a third one.

Dip avocado in flour, shaking off excess.

Dunk in egg blend, then dip in panko and coat them completely.

Put avocado wedges on a baking sheet, and cook them at 400°F until golden, 7 to 8 minutes, turning them after 4 minutes. Season with remaining salt.

While avocado wedges cook, whisk ketchup, mayonnaise, vinegar, turmeric, Sriracha, and pepper to taste in a bowl.

Serve avocado fries with sauce.

NUTRITION FACTS: CALORIES 262KCAL FAT 8 G CARBOHYDRATE11 G PROTEIN 17 G

BUFFALO CAULIFLOWER BITES

 4   30 mins

Ingredients:
3 tbsp. ketchup
2 tbsp. hot sauce
2 egg whites
¾ cup panko (Japanese-style breadcrumbs)
1 lb. cauliflower, cut into florets
1 garlic clove, crushed
1 handful parsley, finely chopped
1/4 tbsp. pepper

Directions:
Whisk together ketchup, hot sauce, parsley, pepper, salt to taste, and egg whites in a bowl until smooth. Add panko to another bowl. Toss together cauliflower florets and ketchup blend in another bowl until covered. Coat the cauliflower with panko mixture.

Cook the cauliflower in the oven at 320°F until colored and firm (around 20 minutes). Serve.

NUTRITION FACTS: CALORIES 125KCAL FAT 4 G CARBOHYDRATE 7 G PROTEIN 8 G

MEDITERRANEAN TOFU SCRAMBLE SNACK

 2   18 mins

Ingredients:
1 tsp. extra virgin olive oil
½ onion, chopped
½ zucchini, chopped
1 cup baby spinach
½ cup halved cherry tomatoes
1 tbsp. sundried tomatoes in oil
4 oz. tofu crumbled

Directions:
Place a pan with oil on medium heat. When hot, add the onion and cook for 5 minutes.

Add zucchini, tomatoes, and spinach. Season with salt and pepper, and cook for 5 minutes until they are soft.

Add tofu and sun-dried tomatoes, finely sliced, and cook 2 minutes. Serve.

NUTRITION FACTS: CALORIES 134KCAL FAT 9 G CARBOHYDRATE 5 G PROTEIN 10 G

CRISPY ONION RINGS WITH SAUCE

 2   🕐 25 mins

Ingredients:
½ cup flour
1 tbsp. smoked paprika
1 egg
1 cup buckwheat breadcrumbs
1 red onion, chopped in 1/2-in
    thick rings
¼ cup low-fat Greek yogurt
2 tbsp. mayonnaise
1 tbsp. ketchup
1 tbsp. Dijon mustard
¼ tbsp. garlic powder
¼ tbsp. paprika
1 cup arugula
1 tsp. extra-virgin olive oil
1 tsp. lime juice

Directions:
Mix flour, smoked paprika, and 1/4 tbsp. of salt in a shallow dish. Delicately beat the egg in another dish, and put breadcrumbs and 1/4 tbsp. of salt in a third one.

Dip onion rings in flour, shaking off excess. Dip in egg, then in breadcrumbs.

Put onion rings in a single layer on a baking sheet, and cook at 375°F for about 10 minutes until crisp, turning them over halfway through cooking.

In the meantime, mix yogurt, mayonnaise, ketchup, mustard, garlic powder, and paprika in a bowl until smooth.

Serve over a simple arugula salad, dressed with 1 tsp. olive oil, 1 tsp. lime juice, salt, and pepper to taste.

NUTRITION FACTS: CALORIES 262KCAL FAT 8 G CARBOHYDRATE 9 G PROTEIN 15 G

THE SCIENCE BEHIND THE SIRTFOOD DIET

The Sirtfood Diet is based on a solid scientific foundation, which is precisely what the Sirtfood diet offers. Let's take a look at the science; I swear you won't get bored!

Scientific Studies on the Skinny Gene

Many studies have indicated that weight variation is greatly influenced by genetics.

Nowadays, lots of research has focused on obesity. A study was conducted by Professor Farooqi and his team to examine the real reason behind why some people remain thin, and others do not.

The study looked at 14,000 participants, of which 1,622 were thin men and women, 1,985 were obese, and over 10,000 people were of average weight. The study compared the DNA of the participants.

The truth is our DNA consists of proteins that are responsible for some particular functions in our bodies. Any kind of change in these genes, genetic variants, can form another protein type, altering the protein's function within the body.

Suppose it's a protein that involves metabolism. In that case, there will be changes in the way our body processes and digests food and even stores the energy.

Furthermore, the team was able to identify some genetic variants that are linked to an increased risk of becoming obese. They were also able to find a novel genetic reason that explains why some are thin (Riveros-McKay et al. 2019).

The impact these genetic variants have on an individual's weight was consolidated in a risk score. It was discovered that thin individuals have a significantly low genetic risk score. The result proved that lean individuals are lean because they possess genes that decrease their chance of becoming obese or overweight.

People believe that genetics is a causal factor of most diseases like cancer, obesity, etc. Genetics make up just 10 percent of the risk factor of these diseases, while the remaining 90 percent is dependent on environmental factors. Surprising right?

The way we sleep, eat, walk, behave, drink, reason, and talk are all factors you control.

In older adults, weight gain is a significant factor in how quickly they age. The fact that your body functions with the 90/10 rule makes it even easier for you to make good use of the genes at your disposal.

There are some genes called famine genes. These are genes that work to assist you in extracting as much energy as they can from the food you consume—thereby giving you the ability to store fat and live through a famine.

While these genes have proven useful for our ancestors at various points in history, they cause us to gain weight more easily for most of us nowadays.

There are also ways in which you can control these genes and activate them as you wish. Even though these genes are a part of you, there are ways you can control them; you have the power to decide how they interact and relate within your body.

Genes Associated with Weight Gain

There are specific genes associated with weight gain that are responsible for how people gain weight unnecessarily, mainly because of their eating habits. Some of these genes include:

The FTO gene

This is the gene that has the strongest link with your body mass index. It's your greatest risk for diabetes and obesity. There's a variant that switches on the gene, and if this variant is present in your body, you will not be able to control the hormone of satiety called leptin. Thus, making you eat unnecessarily. The FTO gene acts as a fat sensor, and people with this kind of gene tend to overeat, especially fatty foods, particularly in childhood. People who share an abnormal gene from both parents weigh more and are at a greater risk of becoming obese. At the same time, people with a normal gene have a lower risk of obesity.

The FTO gene can be switched on with the adequate physical exercise. Ensure you sleep between 7 to 8 hours at night, consume low carbohydrate food, and increase your higher fiber intake. With a proper diet and good lifestyle, your risk of obesity can be reduced.

The Melanocortin 4 Receptor

People born with this gene will consume more snacks, even if they are not hungry. They spend much of their time eating between meals, snacking on cake, chips, and so on. This gene increases cravings for fat.

If you have an increasing urge for a snack, simply learn to eat three times a day. Eat at intervals of four to six hours between each meal, with no snacking in between. Don't rush when eating. Set a boundary for your food consumption so you can easily combat food addiction.

The Adrenergic beta-2 Surface Receptor

This is a different kind of famine gene, and it's associated with the distribution of fat. When this gene is turned on, it can hinder your body fat from breaking down, resulting in a slower metabolic rate, making you store fat. This famine gene can increase your risk of obesity three times over. It can also increase your risk of type 2 diabetes. Also, people with this kind of gene find it challenging to lose weight.

How do you deal with this gene? It's simple. Exercise is one of the possible solutions. Accept that losing weight will be difficult for you so, don't feel bad when you see another person losing weight faster than you. Be disciplined in your eating habits. Eat the right kind of food with the right amount of nutrients. This is a slow and steady mission, so you mustn't rush it.

Weight Loss Regulation

Hypothalamic SIRT1 has been proven to help in weight loss. The hypothalamus is the central weight and energy balance controller. It modulates energy intake and energy consumption through neural inputs from the periphery and direct fluid inputs, which senses the body's energy status.

Leptin, an adipokine, is one of the factors that signal that sufficient energy is stored in the periphery. Leptin plasma levels are favorable for adiposity, suppressing energy intake, and stimulating energy spending.

A prolonged increase in the level of plasma leptin can cause leptin resistance. Leptin resistance, in turn, can prevent the hypothalamus from having access to leptin. This reduces leptin signals transduction in the hypothalamic neurons.

Reduced peripheral energy-sensing by leptin can lead to a positive energy balance and incremental weight gain and adiposity improvements, further exacerbating leptin resistance.

Leptin resistance causes an increase

in adiposity, associated with aging. Similar observations occur in central insulin resistance. Therefore, the improvement of humoral factors in the hypothalamus can prevent progressive weight gains, especially among middle-aged individuals.

SIRT1 is a protein deacetylase, NAD+ dependent with many substrates, such as transcription factors, histones, co-factors, and various enzymes. SIRT1 improves the sensitivity to leptin and insulin by decreasing the levels of several molecules that impair the transduction of leptin and insulin signals. Hypothalamic SIRT1 and NAD+ levels decrease with age.

An increase in the level of SIRT1 has been shown to improve the health in mice and so prevents age-related weight gain. By preventing the loss of age-dependent SIRT1's role in the, there will be a boost in the activity of humoral factors in the hypothalamus and the central energy balance control.

Sirtuins and Metabolic Activity

SIRT1, just like other SIRTUINS, is an NAD+ dependent protein deacetylase associated with cellular metabolism. All sirtuins, including SIRT1, are important for sensing energy status and in protecting against metabolic stress. They coordinate cellular response towards Caloric Restriction (CR) in an organism. SIRT1's diverse location allows cells to easily sense changes in the energy level anywhere in the mitochondria, nucleus, or cytoplasm. They are associated with metabolic health through the deacetylation of several target proteins such as muscles, liver, endothelium, heart, and adipose tissue.

SIRT1, SIRT6, and SIRT7 are localized in the nucleus where they take part in the deacetylation of cytoplasm to influence gene expression epigenetically. SIRT2 is located in the cytosol, while SIRT3, SIRT4, and SIRT5 are located in the mitochondria, where they regulate metabolic enzyme activities and moderate oxidative stress.

SIRT1 aids in mediating the physiological adaptation to diets. Several studies have shown the impact of sirtuins on Caloric Restriction. Sirtuins deacetylase non-histone proteins that define pathways involved during metabolic adaptation when there are metabolic restrictions. Caloric Restriction, on the other hand, causes the induction of expression of SIRT1 in humans. Mutations that lead to loss of function in some sirtuins genes can reduce the effects of caloric restrictions. Sirtuins, therefore, have the functions listed in the following sections.

Regulating the liver

The Liver regulates body glucose homeostasis. During fasting or caloric restriction, glucose levels become low, resulting in a sudden shift in hepatic metabolism to glycogen breakdown and gluconeogenesis to maintain glucose supply and ketone body production to mediate the energy deficit.

Also, during caloric restriction or fasting, muscle activation and liver oxidation of fatty acids are produced during lipolysis in white adipose tissue. For this switch to occur, there are several transcription factors involved to adapt to energy deprivation. SIRT1 intervenes during the metabolic switch to control the energy deficit.

At the initial stage of fasting, that is the post glycogen breakdown phase, there is the production of glucagon by the pancreatic alpha cells to active gluconeogenesis in the Liver through the cyclic amp response element-binding protein (CREB), and CREB regulated transcription coactivator 2 (CRTC2), the coactivator.

During prolonged fasting, the effect is canceled out and replaced by SIRT1 mediated CRTC2 deacetylase, resulting in targeting the coactivator for ubiquitin/proteasome-mediated destruction.

SIRT1, on the other hand, initiates the next

stage of gluconeogenesis through acetylation and activation of peroxisome proliferator-activated receptor coactivator one alpha, which is the coactivator necessary for forkhead box O1. In addition to supporting SIRT1 during gluconeogenesis, coactivator one alpha is required during the mitochondrial biogenesis needed for the liver to accommodate the reduction in energy status. SIRT1 also activates fatty acid oxidation through deacetylation and activation of the nuclear receptor to increase energy production.

SIRT1, when involved in acetylation and the repression of glycolytic enzymes, such as phosphoglycerate mutate 1, can shut down the production of energy through glycolysis. SIRT6, on the other hand, can be used as a co-repressor for hypoxia-inducible Factor 1 Alpha to repress glycolysis. Since SIRT1 can transcriptionally induce SIRT6, sirtuins can coordinate the duration for each fasting phase.

Aside from glucose homeostasis, the liver also takes over lipid and cholesterol homeostasis during fasting. When there are caloric restrictions, the liver's fat and cholesterol synthesis is turned off, while lipolysis in the white adipose tissue commences.

SIRT1, upon fasting, causes the acetylation of steroid regulatory element-binding protein (SREBP) and targets the protein to destroy the ubiquitin-proteasome system.

The result is that fat cholesterol synthesis will be repressed. During the regulation of cholesterol homeostasis, SIRT1 regulates the oxysterol receptor, thereby assisting the reversal of cholesterol transport from peripheral tissue through upregulation of the oxysterol receptor target gene ATP-binding cassette transporter A1 (ABCA1).

Further modulation of the cholesterol regulatory loop can be achieved via the bile acid receptor, necessary for the biosynthesis of cholesterol catabolic and bile acid pathways. SIRT6 also participates in regulating cholesterol levels by repressing the expression and post-translational cleavage of SREBP1/2 into the active form. Furthermore, in the circadian regulation of metabolism, SIRT1 participates through regulating the cellular circadian clock.

Mitochondrial SIRT3 is crucial in the oxidation of fatty acid in mitochondria. Fasting or caloric restrictions can result in the up-regulation of activities and levels of SIRT3 to aid fatty acid oxidation through deacetylation of long-chain specific acyl-CoA dehydrogenase. SIRT3 can also cause the activation of ketogenesis and the urea cycle in the liver.

SIRT1 also acts in the metabolic regulation in the muscle and white adipose tissue. Fasting causes an increase in the level of SIRT1, leading to the deacetylation of coactivator one alpha, which causes the activation of genes responsible for fat oxidation.

The reduction in energy level also activates AMPK, which will activate the expression of coactivator one alpha. The combined effects of the two processes will increase mitochondrial biogenesis and fatty acid oxidation in the muscle.

Sirtuins, Muscles, and Oxidative Capacity

The expression of sirtuin in the muscle is affected by physical exercise, which controls cellular antioxidant system changes, mitochondrial biogenesis, and oxidative metabolism.

Skeletal muscles are involved in force and movement and engaged in endocrine activities by their ability to secrete cytokines and transcription factors into the bloodstream, thereby controlling other organs' functions. Furthermore, skeletal muscle is a metabolically active tissue that plays a vital role in maintaining the body's metabolism.

The skeletal muscle makes up about 40% of the entire weight of the body. The insulin-stimulated uptake of glucose and the main energy-consuming lipid catabolism is mainly at this site. For skeletal muscle, metabolic flexibility is essential to preserve physiological processes and metabolic homeostasis.

It determines the ability to switch from glucose to lipid oxidation. Advances in the understanding of the molecular mechanisms underlying skeletal muscle activity are a therapeutic benefit. Sirtuins' roles have been widely investigated in skeletal muscle, specifically concerning their role in controlling glucose and lipid metabolism, insulin functions and sensitivity, and mitochondrial biogenesis.

Cellular metabolic stress results from physical exercise, which affects the sirtuins. The most studied sirtuins in this respect are SIRT1 and SIRT3: SIRT1 is localized in the nucleus while SIRT3, in the mitochondria. SIRT3 is more expressed in type I muscle fiber.

One study showed that mouse skeletal muscle SIRT3 reacted to the six-week voluntary exercise dynamically to coordinate the downstream molecular response (Palacios et al., 2009). The result also showed that movement increases SIRT3 protein, CREB, coactivator one alpha, and citrate synthesis activity.

The downregulation of CREB, AMP-activated protein kinase (AMPK) phosphorylation, and the mRNA of PGC-1⊠ are all symptoms of SIRT3 knockout. This shows that these key cellular molecules are essential for SIRT3 to carry out the biological signals effectively.

Palacios et al. discovered that SIRT3 responds to exercise dynamically to enhance muscular energy homeostasis through AMPK and PGC-1⊠. Voluntary exercise causes an increase in the SIRT3 content of skeletal muscle. Muscle Immobility can, therefore, lead to the downregulation of SIRT3.

Furthermore, SIRT1 protein content and PGC-1 in the muscle tends to increase with exercise. Bayod et al. (2012) reported that SIRT1 protein content and PGC-1 in rat's muscle increased after 36 weeks of treadmill training and enhancement in antioxidant defenses.

There's an increase in ATP demand during exercise, leading to increased NAD+ level and NAD+/NADH ratio. The result is an increase in the substrate for SIRT1 and SIRT3. SIRT3 is responsible for the increased ATP production and a reduction in protein synthesis in the mitochondria.

The ATP produced activates and deacetylases tricarboxylic acid (TCA) enzymes, electron transport chain, and ⊠-oxidation, which maximizes the availability of reducing equivalents for ATP production. SIRT1, on the other hand, responds to exercise by contributing to mitochondrial biogenesis via independent mechanisms.

In summary, strenuous exercise activates SIRT1, which enhances biogenesis and mitochondrial oxidative capacity.

Furthermore, repeated sessions of strenuous exercise will activate both SIRT1 and SIRT3, which in turn start ATP production and the mitochondrial antioxidant function.

APPENDIX C - FREQUENTLY ASKED QUESTIONS

Below is included a list of the most frequently asked questions and their answers.

DO I EXERCISE DURING PHASE 1?

Regular exercise is one of the best things you can do for your health. Doing some moderate exercise can improve your weight loss and well-being. As a general rule, during the Sirtfood Diet's first seven days, we advise you to maintain your average exercise and physical activity level. We suggest staying in your usual comfort zone, as prolonged or overly intense training can simply put too much stress on the body during this time. Check your body. There's no need to force yourself to do more exercise during Phase 1; instead, let the sirtfoods do the hard work.

I AM SLIM — CAN I FOLLOW THE DIET?

For anyone underweight, we do not recommend Phase 1 of the Sirtfood Diet as you don't need to lose any more weight. Calculating your body mass index or BMI is a safe way to understand if you are underweight. You can easily calculate this by using one of the numerous online BMI calculators, as long as you know your height and weight. If your BMI is 18.5 or less, we do not suggest embarking on phase 1 of the diet. We would also advise caution if your BMI is between 18.5 and 20 because following the diet could mean that your BMI falls below 18.5. While many people strive to be super-skinny, the fact is that being underweight may have a detrimental effect on your health, leading to a weakened immune system, an increased risk of osteoporosis (weakened bones), and fertility issues. What you could do is follow Phase 3 — Transition and use the recipes in the book to create your Meal Plan. You should follow the guidelines of Phase 3, as it does not include caloric restriction but helps you set up a diet rich in sirtfoods.

I AM OBESE — IS THE SIRTFOOD DIET RIGHT FOR ME?

Of course! Join the thousands of people who already tried the diet and lost weight. You will reap considerable improvements in your well-being, thanks to sirtuin activation. Being obese increases the risk of many chronic health problems, yet these are the very illnesses that sirtfoods will help you avoid.

I REACHED MY TARGET WEIGHT, AND DON'T WANT TO LOSE ANY MORE — DO I STOP EATING SIRTFOODS?

First of all, congratulations on your success! With sirtfoods, even if you have seen great success, it doesn't stop when you reach your goal. While we do not recommend further calorie restriction, your diet should still provide ample sirtfoods. The great thing about sirtfoods is that they are a lifestyle. In terms of weight control, the best way to think of them as a way to help get the body into the weight and shape it was meant to be and stay there. They will continue to work to maintain your weight and keep you looking fantastic and feeling great.

I TAKE MEDICATION — IS IT OK TO FOLLOW THE DIET?

The Sirtfood Diet is ideal for most people. Still, due to its powerful effects on fat burning and well-being, it can alter the processes of certain diseases and the medication plan recommended by your doctor.

If you suffer from a significant health condition, take prescription medications, or have any reasons to think about going on a diet, we recommend that you speak to your doctor about it. Likely, you could profoundly benefit from the Sirtfood Diet, but you should check with your physician first.

WILL I GET A HEADACHE OR TIRED FEEL DURING PHASE 1?

This diet can include mild headaches or tiredness, but these effects are slight and short-lived. Of course, if the symptoms are severe or give you cause for concern, seek medical advice promptly. Occasional mild symptoms will quickly resolve, and within a few days, most people have a renewed sense of energy, vigor, and well-being.

SHOULD I REPEAT PHASES 1, 2, AND 3?

You can repeat Phase 1 if you feel you need to lose more weight or need a health boost. To ensure no long-term adverse effects of calorie restriction appear, you should wait at least a month before repeating it. Most people need to repeat it no more than once every three months and to see excellent results. Instead, if you have gone off course, need some fine-tuning, or want a little more sirtfood pressure, we suggest that you repeat Phase 2 and 3 as often as you want, as these are about developing lifelong eating habits. Remember, the Sirtfood Diet's beauty is that it doesn't require you to feel like you're endlessly on a diet. Instead, it's the foundation for developing positive lifelong dietary changes that will create a lighter, leaner, healthier you.

DOES THE SIRTFOOD DIET HAVE ENOUGH FIBER?

Many sirtfoods are naturally rich in fiber. Onions, endives, and walnuts are notable sources, with buckwheat and Medjool dates standing out too, meaning The Sirtfood Diet is not short in the fiber department. Even during Phase 1, when food consumption is reduced, most dieters will still consume an acceptable fiber quantity, particularly if recipes are selected from the menu containing buckwheat, beans, and lentils. However, for others known to be susceptible to intestinal problems such as constipation without high fiber intake, a suitable fiber supplement may be considered during Phase 1, especially days 1 to 3, which should be discussed with your health care professional.

CAN I EAT WHAT I WANT ONCE I EAT PLENTY OF SIRTFOODS AND STILL SEE RESULTS?

One of the main reasons why the Sirtfood Diet works so well in the long term is that it encourages good food rather than demonizing mediocre food. Exclusion diets just aren't effective long-term. Processed foods high in sugars and fats decrease sirtuin activity in the body, thus reducing the benefits of sirtfood consumption. However, if you stay focused on eating a diet rich in sirtfoods, you will end up consuming much less garbage than the average person, and, as a result, you will feel happy and fulfilled and have less appetite for certain refined foods. If you sometimes indulge in these refined foods, don't worry about it — the strength of sirtfoods, the rest of the time, will ensure that you are still reaping the benefits.

CAN MY FAMILY JOIN ME IN THIS JOURNEY AND EAT THE SAME MEALS I PREPARE FOR MYSELF?

Of course, they can, and while their support will be of great help for you, they will also benefit from the sirtuin's anti-oxidant effect. As a result, the whole family will feel great in no time. Just a quick reminder about portions: remember that you may need to adapt them to different needs. Men may require larger quantities, while kids could eat much less. As long as the meals include plenty of sirtfoods, it will be ok. Of course, coffee and wine are to avoid with children, while spicy meals with chili are already excluded from this version of the Sirtfood Diet because of their effect on menopause symptoms.

Your honest review of this book is very much appreciated. Your feedback is important to me, and it will help other readers decide whether to read the book too.

Thank you! Kate Hamilton

Made in the USA
Coppell, TX
09 November 2021